The Skinny

How to fit into your little black dress forever

The eat-what-you-want way
to lose weight and keep it off

Melissa Clark & Robin Aronson

Foreword by Darwin Deen, MD

Meredith® Books   Des Moines, Iowa

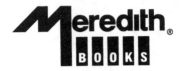

Meredith Books
1716 Locust Street
Des Moines, Iowa 50309–3023
meredithbooks.com

Printed in the United States of America.

First Edition.
Library of Congress Control Number: 2006930038
ISBN-13: 978-0-696-23242-8

See your doctor first.
This diet and fitness book is designed to provide helpful information on the
subjects addressed. This book is sold with the understanding that the authors
and publisher are not rendering medical, health, or other personal services. The
suggestions for specific exercise routines, foods, and lifestyle recommendations
are not intended to replace medical advice or treatment by your physician. All
questions and concerns regarding your health, metabolism, weight, nutrition, and
physical activity should be directed to your physician, particularly if you have any
health problems or medical problems (including if you are pregnant or lactating).
All reasonable attempts have been made to include the most recent and factual
research and medical reports regarding exercise and nutrition. However, there is
no guarantee that future research, particularly human studies, will not change the
information presented here. Individual needs vary, and no nutrition or exercise
program will meet everyone's needs. Be sure to consult your physician prior to
following any of the suggestions presented in this book and also before changing
your diet or exercise routine. You should rely on your physician's advice regarding
whether the suggestions presented in this book are appropriate for you, and
you should rely on your physician to establish your weight goal. The authors
and publisher disclaim all liability associated with the recommendations and
guidelines set forth in this book. Further, the Internet addresses in this book were
accurate at the time of printing.

for Mara

Acknowledgments

Thank you to Linda Cunningham, Stephanie Karpinske, Som Inthalangsy, and everyone at Meredith for bringing our vision of *The Skinny* to life. Thanks to Carrie Bachman and Amy Nichols for helping us get *The Skinny* message out there. This project would not have gotten off the ground without Janis Donnaud, our agent and best critic. She is our Tim Gunn (please say you watch *Project Runway*), and when she says, "Make it work, people," we do.

Melissa: This book never would have happened without Robin's enthusiasm, talent, pregnancy, and subsequent weight gain and loss—not to mention it was her idea to write it in the first place. Thanks, Robin, for all of the above, and much, much more. Thanks to Sarah Huck, my fabulous recipe tester, for putting up with the lean as well as the fat, and a lot of long hours. Thanks to my parents, Rita and Julian Clark, for teaching me about the pleasures of the table from a very early age, and to my sister Amy, another writer in the family, for understanding what deadlines mean, and helping me stick to them (sort of). A very belated thanks to Stacy Nelson, who convinced me to start running when I was 17 with these words: "Think of it as 20 minutes a day you'll spend taking care of your body and getting skinny." She was right! Thanks to Alice Feiring, my discerning travel buddy and wine mentor, with whom I've tossed out as many cookies, pastries, and bottles of wine as we've shared together. Only the very best makes the cut with Alice. Thanks to Frank Bruni for being so smart, so savvy, and such a supportive friend, and for feeding me more than I can ever finish. And, thanks to Daniel Gercke, who knows why.

Robin: I must thank you, Melissa, for being an excellent friend, a superior collaborator, and something of an inspiration. My cousin and dear friend Cara Cohen Hiller also has been an inspiration (even if she doesn't know it). She is one of my favorite dining companions and one of the pickiest eaters I've ever encountered. She really eats just what she wants. Many thanks, as always, to Natalie Dohrmann, Sarah Hill, Dorothy Novick Kenney, Nicole Marwell, Elsie Stern, and Mary Recine Struthers. My family is chock full of good cooks and happy eaters. Thanks to Louis, Ami, Caroline, Melissa, Isaac, and Goldie Aronson for making big holiday meals lively good fun. My parents Edward and Myrna Aronson always told me I could do whatever I set my mind to doing—except, of course, when it came to helping my mom cook. No one helps Myrna cook (cleaning up, now that's a different story). Thanks for all those meals and for teaching me about the importance of eating together as a family. And then there's my own family. David Stone, my husband, could not possibly be more supportive of me, my writing, and my cookie baking. My kids, Helen and Elliot, well, what can I say? Helen's delight in blueberries, Elliot's disgust at bananas—every day they show me what it is to discern and fully enjoy the flavors and pleasures of life.

Foreword
by Darwin Deen, MD

Sometimes it seems as if everyone in America is struggling with their weight, and it is almost true. National statistics demonstrate that more than half of Americans are already overweight. Surveys also show that many people are trying to lose weight—yet overall we keep gaining weight. The diet industry earns billions of dollars each year selling "miracle" supplements, programs, and remedies with no science behind them, and diet books seem to proliferate like mushrooms. The updated 2005 U.S. Dietary Guidelines finally abandoned overly simplistic messages such as "maintain a healthy weight." Instead, the guidelines now advise people to focus on reducing calories and increasing physical activity to achieve lasting weight control. However, when it comes to finding a program that you can live with, it's not that easy.

Into this chaotic situation, Melissa Clark and Robin Aronson seek to inject a little sanity. Written by a food writer and a health writer, *The Skinny* is a well-thought-out book that provides solid advice that's presented in an easily accessible style. *The Skinny* is not another fad diet book. Because the authors advocate eating what you want when you want it, you can avoid the feelings of deprivation that so many people experience when dieting, and that eventually cause them to fail.

Presented in part as a dialogue between two friends, *The Skinny* invites the reader into their conversations, and it helps us discover what to eat and how to eat to avoid the necessity of constant dieting. The authors espouse "little black dress behavior" which calls for a return to commonsense and lays out a simple program composed of easy-to-follow rules that will help readers in their weight loss and weight-maintenance efforts. The book is entertaining as well as informative and provides clear and helpful tips that can be implemented on an everyday basis. The benefit of two different viewpoints from women who have different lifestyles, different metabolisms, and unique eating preferences helps demonstrate that these rules can be applied regardless of who you are.

The authors advise portion control and yet recognize how difficult that is in the American marketplace. Whether it is buying in bulk at the local supermarket to save money, purchasing extra-large servings because they appear cost-effective, or ordering à la carte in family-style restaurants where the dinner plates are the size of serving platters, we have come to believe the message that bigger is better. Understanding how to give yourself what your body needs (not *wants*, just needs) is clearly outlined in this book. *The Skinny* helps you figure out how to eat to maintain your weight or lose weight, and it gives you the tools to balance what you eat with your physical activity. This is a critical point because regardless of what you eat—carbohydrates, proteins, or fats—if you don't expend (burn) as many calories as you consume (take in), you won't lose (or even maintain your) weight. Unfortunately in this day and age, with the increases in almost all portion sizes, the majority of us are eating and drinking more calories than necessary without realizing it.

I have dozens of patients who have successfully lost weight on low-carbohydrate regimens only to abandon the dietary discipline because they crave pasta or potatoes. Soon thereafter they are disappointed to discover that all their weight-loss efforts have been undone. Melissa and Robin help the reader to break out of this endless yo-yo cycle of dieting and binging. They show you instead how to eat sensibly when you can— and ignore sensible eating when you must.

Their philosophy is liberating. The tools offered in this book, including self-reflection and visualization, can be used by anyone and will make you a happier, healthier person, no matter what you weigh. The recipe section contains easy-to-prepare yet remarkably tasty fare. They use simple preparation methods and ingredients, and they are respectful of the time that food preparation takes—even offering many ideas for altering basic takeout food to make it healthier, lower in calories, and more appealing. So enjoy *The Skinny*—and getting into and staying in your "little black dress."

Darwin Deen, MD
Chief, Undergraduate Medical Education
Professor, Department of Family and Social Medicine, Albert Einstein
 College of Medicine
Associate Professor, Department of Epidemiology and Population Health

Dr. Darwin Deen is a nationally recognized family physician who has been studying and teaching nutrition for almost 30 years. Dr. Deen currently practices family medicine and nutrition in the Bronx, New York, where he has been taking care of patients for more than 20 years.

Contents

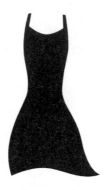

The perfect little black dress.

Every woman has one. The sexy number she just had to buy and probably paid way too much for. The designer frock she pulls off the hanger whenever she has a hot date, a see-and-be-seen cocktail party, or a fancy dinner. It's the off-the-rack equivalent of a best friend: dependable, flattering when and where she deserves it, a partner in crime. It's the ubiquitous clothing item that's ready to support her through thick and thin. Preferably thin.

And there's the rub. The staying thin. We've all had that horrifying, "Did the dry cleaner shrink my dress?" moment. The flash when you realize that the chapter in your life when you could eat whatever you wanted and not gain weight is, unfortunately, over. And now you have to do something about those extra pounds.

But what's your plan? Are you going to give up ice cream for a month? Turn your back on your true love, the chocolate chip cookie? Refuse to sip another cocktail? Ban the bread basket and live on bacon and eggs? No. Because you've tried those tricks already, and even though you lost some weight, you always put it back on.

That's because at some point you remembered how good pizza and guacamole-dunked tortilla chips taste. Or you couldn't come up with a good reason not to have the brownie that chatted you up while you waited to pay for your nice green salad. Before you know it, it's so long, little black dress. Hope to see you again soon. Thus the ineffective and torturous dieting cycle begins anew.

But not this time. Because you are about to embark on an eating adventure that will last a lifetime. *The Skinny* offers you an approach to meals that will keep you not only looking fabulous but also feeling satisfied with what you eat—because no foods are banned. After all, food is one of life's great joys, and we say: Dig in.

The Skinny's not-so-skinny beginning

We—Melissa and Robin—decided to write *The Skinny* because we like to eat. But we don't like being told what to eat and what not to eat; we want to make those decisions for ourselves. Sure, being told exactly what to have at each meal works for short-term weight loss, but keeping the weight off for months and years? That requires a better strategy. We know because both of us have been there and done that on the weight loss and weight control front.

We're longtime friends who lead very different lives. Melissa does the single, sophisticated-girl-about-town thing, and Robin does the family thing. We started talking about how to eat— conversations that turned into *The Skinny*—a year after Robin had twins. Robin was struggling to lose the last 20 pounds of pregnancy weight, but the only thing she knew to do about her weight was complain. To her size 2 friend, Melissa. Really, Robin whined, how could she possibly diet when that would mean being food-deprived on top of being sleep-deprived?

Then one day Robin decided to stop complaining and ask Melissa for advice. Why Melissa? Because she's a food writer

ROBIN'S LITTLE BLACK DRESS MOMENT

It was late in the summer when my twins were 10 months old, and I had to go to a fancy-ish cocktail party. I opened my closet about two weeks before the party and held up my trusted, go-to little black dress. With one look I knew it was not an option. But because I'm either eternally optimistic or a glutton for punishment, I tried it on. And then tried it off. Quickly. And then I didn't think about the party again until the day before, when I ran out and got something Just Fine for not a lot of money. I thought I could wear the dress again if I had to, but I really didn't want to have to. I knew my complaining wasn't helping me lose weight, even though I wasn't quite sure why not. Why couldn't I actualize weight loss by bitching about weight gain?

and a size 2. Because she is able to give advice with attitude but without condescension. And because Melissa once weighed (a lot) more, but she lost the weight when she was 23 and has kept it off—all while building a career centered on food and going out to eat.

As a food writer, Melissa not only eats in restaurants most nights of the week, but when she's at home, she's writing cookbooks with some of the best chefs in the world. Big names like Daniel Boulud and David Bouley. Pastry chefs such as Claudia Fleming and Bill Yosses. (We should mention that Melissa has an overactive sweet tooth.) And when you write a cookbook, you cook all the food in it. And then you eat it—at least some of it. You have to. It's your job. Every day.

Most people Melissa meets—not just desperate new moms looking for a way back to their pre-pregnancy weight—ask her how she maintains such a sleek figure while eating at some of the best restaurants in the world with enviable regularity.

Robin paid close attention to what Melissa had to say about eating. Melissa said that no food is forbidden. (Because of her job, Melissa will eat anything, and she means *anything*.) But all foods are subject to limits. She said that when she really enjoys what she's eating, she doesn't feel deprived. She makes sure to include fruits and vegetables with every meal, even if that means ordering a salad on the side of her foie gras. Then, of course, she talked about exercise. (Yes, do it.)

Robin followed Melissa's advice and started paying attention to what she ate. On Melissa's plan, to her surprise, Robin never thought, "I can't have this peanut butter cup" or "I will never again eat a bagel." Because no food was outlawed, the plan didn't feel like a diet. Instead it felt like a fresh, new approach, which soon morphed into new eating habits: more fruit for snacks, loads of veggies at mealtime, smaller portions, and the (guilt-free) cookie that Robin always needs at the end of the day.

And a weird thing happened. Instead of losing the last 20 pregnancy pounds, she lost 30. Robin's now the thinnest she's been since college. The weight isn't coming back on. And people started asking how she did it.

So, here's how. It's life on *The Skinny*.

MELISSA'S MUSINGS ON GENES AND JEANS

Not a week goes by without someone—neighbor, colleague, chef—asking me how I stay so thin as a food writer. Most of them assume I just have one of those hyperactive, ectomorphic metabolisms, meaning I can put it away like a football player yet keep the figure of a cheerleader.

The fact is, until I figured out how to live *The Skinny* life, I was trapped in that miserable cycle of gaining and losing those same 5, 10, even 35 pounds. I come from a long line of zaftig food lovers, going back as far as my family photos can attest. My parents are passionate eaters who between them have gained and lost more than 100 pounds over the decades. (I do not exaggerate.) My sister, too, struggles with her weight, battling anywhere between 5 and 60 pounds. Simply put, my genes are just not those of a skinny girl.

But thanks to my life on *The Skinny*, my jeans are.

This is not a discrete, two-week diet plan. (Although to get you started, we do include a "2-Week Meal Plan," page 227.) Rather, *The Skinny* is a new way to think about the food you love, the food you must have, and the food you eat all the time.

It's an approach that balances a life of eating smart and lean with a life of eating rich (fried chicken, cookies, potato chips, ice cream, whatever). Because we all agree it's impossible to give up the good stuff for good. Always ordering healthy, steamed vegetables instead of General Tso's chicken? That's a huge drag. No one can live that way for her whole life.

The Skinny shows you how to mix the whole-fat with the fat-free, the scallion pancakes with the broccoli in garlic sauce. *The Skinny* refuses to make you spend every cocktail party mooning over mini burgers and bacon-wrapped scallops while nursing a plain carrot stick and glumly sipping sparkling water. (On *The Skinny*, we say choose your favorite three hors d' oeuvres and eat one of each, savoring every bite. Then follow up with the carrots—but with a little dip. Jeez.) This is a way you can eat for your whole life.

You can eat *The Skinny* way whether you're making a quick dinner at home or eating out on a hot date with a new prospect or a longtime love. You can eat this way in any of the situations where eating "light" seems a little outré: the holiday meal, your weekly lunch at the burger joint with work pals, the fancy dinner with your significant other's boss, the reunion dinner with an old friend with whom you always eat (ate) big. In other words, in *The Skinny*, we give you a new way to think about what you want to eat, what you need to eat, and what you crave.

The Skinny recipes

Eating lots of fruits and veggies is at the core of *The Skinny*. After all, produce gives the biggest nutritional bang for your caloric buck. Fruits and vegetables reduce the risk of a host of diseases, sate your hunger, and make your skin glow. Now really, what could be bad about eating more of them?

So Melissa created 75 simple yet delicious recipes that will help you build healthy eating habits. These recipes give you a range of produce-based cuisine, so you won't be burdened with trying to come up with something new to do with green beans. You'll never again make a peanut butter and jelly sandwich for want of ideas or time. (For just plain want, however, no problem. Have the PB&J! That's exactly what *The Skinny* is about.)

For us eating is not about guilt. It's about pleasure and good health, decadence, and restraint. We like to be a little good and a little naughty and a lot happy—happy with our food, our clothes, our shoes, ourselves, our bodies. Living life on *The Skinny* is how we do it.

Chapter 1

Happy Skinny

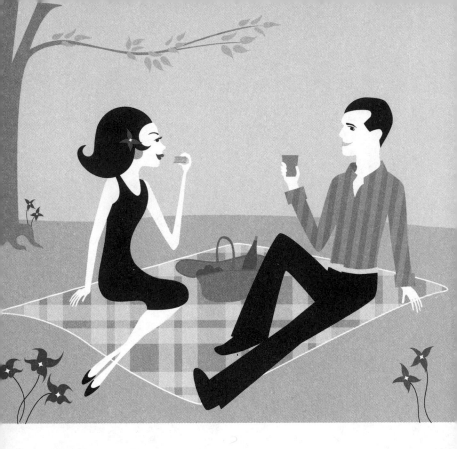

What is Happy Skinny?

According to the dictionary, "skinny" is an adjective meaning thin. It also means "the truth about something," so here are three truths about being thin:

- "Thin" is a state of mind that, for better or worse, generally translates to "I feel good about my body."

- Feeling good about your body often translates into feeling good in general.

- Being thin does not make life meaningful. Likewise, food does not give life meaning, but it does give pleasure. Let's enjoy.

Enjoying your food and enjoying your body: That's how we define Happy Skinny. It's not about dress size. It's about experiencing pleasure and being comfortable in your own skin. What does it take to reach Happy Skinny? It's different for everyone, but here are some things we think are important for the journey.

The state of mind thing

You may be saying, "Sure, 'thin' is a state of mind, but it's also a state where I can wear my 'skinny jeans,' a state where my little black dress is a little littler."

Point taken. But how many times have you gotten on the scale and if it reads two pounds more than yesterday you feel bad, and if it reads two pounds less you feel good? Can anyone see those two pounds? No.

Because we're dynamic, ever-changing creatures, our weight fluctuates throughout each day. We weigh a little more in the middle of the day and a little less in the morning. (And maybe we shouldn't get on the scale so much that we know this.) We haven't morphed into different beings by noon; we've just eaten breakfast and maybe a snack.

Of course the world we live in is not kind when it comes to weight. It is competitive and demanding, and every form of media tells us that when you are actually thin (not simply living happily in a thin state of mind), your life is better and you are better. You show the world that you have discipline and restraint. You must be successful and happy and loved. Right?

Not necessarily. You are not a better or worse person depending on the number on the scale. Weighing more or less is not inherently good or bad, aside from the health aspects. Nor will weighing less solve all your problems or make you a happier, more successful person.

Whether you decide to lose 5 pounds or 40, the decision has to be yours alone. Don't make the decision because it's what you imagine your family or the person who makes your heart race wants. It must be because it's what you want.

Five good reasons to try The Skinny

1. If you're carrying around more than 10 extra pounds (or less, if you're fairly short), you'll feel stronger, more mobile, and overall physically better weighing less.

2. Your clothes will fit better, so you'll feel better in them, and you'll project that good feeling when you go out in the world.

3. You'll like to look at yourself in the mirror, even naked, without sucking it in too much.

4. You'll know you can lose weight if and when you want to, and you'll revel in that accomplishment.

5. You'll have a good reason to go clothes shopping.

Five bad reasons to try The Skinny

1. You want to fit back into your cheerleading outfit/prom dress from high school. (Give up the ghost.)

2. You think you have to be skinny to wear the latest fashions. (Even size 2 Melissa can't pull off most of today's fashions. No one wants to be skeletal-model-skinny anyway.)

3. You think people will like you better if you're thinner.

4. You think your weight is what's stopping you from personal or career success.

5. You think losing weight will fix all your problems.

The body in your little black dress

Inside every little black dress, every chic sheath, and every pair of Yanuk jeans, there's a body. Bodies are lovely things, full of power and sensation, ready for anything. And yet it's probably fair to say that everyone has things about her body that she

WHY GET ON *THE SKINNY* IF YOU'RE ALREADY SKINNY?

Life on *The Skinny* is a long-term proposition. We're talking about committing to a life in which you eat better because you eat what you want (and you eat a diet built on lots of fruits and vegetables). Living on *The Skinny* means you learn how to tuck into the good and steer clear of the bad. And that's the best and easiest way to maintain your healthy, Happy Skinny weight over the long haul.

appreciates more, and things she appreciates less. But there's no denying that our bodies are our very own, and no one else will ever appreciate them as completely, complexly, and deeply as we do ourselves. And so it's worth treating our bodies with respect and care. Part of respecting your body is not loathing it because you think you need to lose a few pounds or because of how your stomach looked in the skirt you tried on the other day (and that certainly could be the fault of the cut of the skirt and not at all the fault of your belly).

The Skinny on healthy weight

By now you've probably heard a thing or three about the Body Mass Index (BMI), which measures body fatness based on height and weight. (To calculate your BMI, see page 243.) The "healthy" range on the BMI scale—the weight range that correlates to a lower risk of developing heart disease, diabetes, and possibly some cancers—is 18.5 to 24.9. Some nutrition experts argue that this range should be cut off at 22 instead of 24.9 because it's above 22 that levels of weight-related diseases start to rise.

The truth is that while BMI is a helpful tool many people can use to figure out their healthy weight range, it's not useful for everyone. It's not an

MELISSA'S HAPPY SKINNY STATS

Height: 5'6"

Current/ideal weight: 111 to 113 pounds

Highest weight: 148 pounds

Weight loss: 36 pounds at age 23

Exercise: At least four times a week, ideally six. A combination of running, stair machine, yoga, Pilates, free weights, and walking quickly all over the city.

My most favorite body parts:
Clavicle. Mine protrudes delicately and calls attention to my bust, which doesn't call for attention on its own.

Hair. It's a lovely shade of strawberry blond and is just thick enough to curl or straighten as I command it with blow dryer and brush.

The mole on my cheek. Combined with my reddish hair, it makes me feel like Ginger from *Gilligan's Island*. Very glam, that mole.

My least favorite body parts:
Outer thighs. Yes, even skinny girls get cellulite, and I've got it.

Butt. I have a flat, bony butt. Even if I gained 5 pounds, it would go to my belly, not my butt.

Teeth. They're yellowish, despite numerous applications of bleaching strips.

oracle. Because it was created for the widest possible group—everyone—it cannot take into account individual variations, such as your body's fat-to-muscle ratio, your own personal genetics, and your lifestyle.

ROBIN'S HAPPY SKINNY STATS

Height: 5'7" (and a quarter!)

Current/ideal weight: 132 pounds

Weight before _The Skinny:_ 140 to 148 pounds

Highest weight: 202 pounds (when I was pregnant)

Weight loss: 71 pounds after having twins

How long it took: 40 pounds in 3 weeks; 31 pounds in 11 months

Exercise: Yoga, swimming, biking, walking, schlepping up and down the stairs, and playing with my kids.

My most favorite body parts: **Nose.** It's straight and kind of pointy, but I think it's a good nose.

Waist. My waist has always been tapered, even after having twins.

Thighs. I have big thigh muscles. In yoga class, they feel like they're strong enough to hold up the world.

My least favorite body parts: **Belly.** A girl's flat stomach is never the same after it's been asked to hold two babies at once.

Knees. Don't ask.

Thighs. It's such a cliché. I either love my big, strong thighs or hate them.

You could have a BMI of 19, which is way down at the low end of the healthy range. But if you keep your weight low by smoking, well, it's fairly obvious that your weight no longer correlates to a lower risk of heart disease or cancer.

On the flip side, you could have a BMI on the higher end of the range. But if you exercise regularly (so you have lots of muscle, which weighs more than fat), eat mostly fresh foods, avoid a lot of processed, fried, or otherwise unhealthy foods, and are generally healthy (let's say we're defining that by having normal blood pressure and cholesterol levels), your long-term health risks are lower than your BMI might indicate. (For the record, Tom Cruise has a high BMI.)

Remember, BMI is just one way to figure out a healthy weight range, and weight range is only one part of the good health picture. If you're physically active and make reasonable lifestyle choices, from a health perspective it kind of doesn't matter what you weigh or, more to the point, what your BMI is.

You know the weight that is most stable and consistent for you, where you feel comfortable, and where you're not driving yourself mad thinking about that brownie you had for a midday snack.

Of course, you can be pretty healthy and pretty fit and still want to drop a few because you want your little Tocca dress to be a little swishier when you prance out the door. That's where *The Skinny* comes in. Eat reasonably, eat what you love, and feel fabulous.

THE CREEP (OR WHEN 2 POUNDS IS MORE THAN JUST 2 POUNDS)

It's fair to say that when it comes to weight, we all have a healthy, happy zone at which we feel our best. For some women—like Melissa—that range is 2 pounds. For others—like Robin—it's more like 3 to 5 pounds. Regardless of the exact number, if you find that you're consistently at the top of your zone for a couple of weeks during your regular weigh-ins, consider scaling back what you're eating in order to drop back down to your sweet spot.

Why? Because if you don't, over time those 1 or 2 pounds will add up. Take the holidays, for example. Gaining 1 to 2 pounds during the last six weeks of the year isn't the end of the world. After all, sometimes the best way to deal with your annoying cousin Irv is to simply nod your head while your mouth is full of pecan pie. And what's a pound or 2? It's not a lot, relatively speaking.

But if you don't drop those 2 pounds, and if you continue to gain a pound or 2 every holiday season, then over five years you've gained 5 to 10 pounds. We call this The Creep.

It's a hell of a lot easier to drop those first 2 pounds than get rid of the 10. So we say, "Defend yourself against The Creep!"

The exception: Of course, a woman will gain a big chunk of weight when she gets pregnant. She's supposed to. And losing it is tough because your body changes and, let's face it, you don't have a lot of time to think about what you've just eaten or when you're going to get to your next yoga class. Still, after a year or so it's time to take a step back and try to reestablish what your healthy weight zone is. It may or may not be the same as it was before the baby, but you've got to be able to recognize it and feel good about it.

How much exercise does it take to be Happy Skinny? (Try how little.)

There are many good reasons to exercise. It helps manage stress. It helps you maintain or lose weight. (We would say, "It burns calories," but we don't believe in counting calories; see page 26.) Most important, once you find the exercise that's right for you, physical activity feels good and will make you happy.

For all these reasons, everyone should exercise regularly. But to simply improve your health, you only need to be reasonably active. You may ask, "What's that?" A reasonable question. "Reasonably active" means you move around more than just walking to the bathroom and to your car, or tossing and turning in bed at night. And believe it or not, by "move around" we're not only talking about exercise in a gym.

If on a typical day you really do only walk from your house to your car to the office, add 10 minutes of walking to your day by parking at the far end of the lot when you go to the office, the mall, and the supermarket. Or take the stairs. Or dance around your living room for 10 minutes. Or do 20 minutes of housework: vacuuming, dusting, scurrying around, and putting things away. (This is theoretically easy to do if you have small children because

ROBIN ON THE SWEET SMELL OF SWEAT

I'm no athlete. When I was a kid, I was always picked last for team sports. I'd run the other way if a softball floated my way. I scored a touchdown once. For the other team. But just because I have a checkered athletic history doesn't mean I don't like to exercise. In fact, I've learned over the years that I pretty much love it.

I wandered into a yoga class at my gym one day when I wasn't in the mood for spinning. I was immediately hooked. Obsessed. Yoga changed my life.

I thank my lucky stars that my parents sent me to summer camp. Not only because it was fun (and sometimes I was picked second to last for team sports), but also because it was there that I learned to swim. Now I go swimming as often as I can. It makes me ridiculously happy to be immersed in water.

Of course sometimes a swim is just a swim, and a yoga class is just a yoga class, and there's nothing transporting about it. But when a swim or a class is pretty damn good, it's just great. All this to say, when it comes to exercise, find your bliss.

you'll have a lot to put away at the end of the day. Then again if you have small children, at the end of the day when you would normally scurry around and clean up, you may want to curl up in a ball and nap for 20 minutes instead.) Move your body just a little more, and it will be happy. And if you add in sustained exercise—we aim for at least 30 minutes three to four times a week—you'll eventually be Happy Skinny too.

The Takeaway

- Happy Skinny means figuring out how to feel good in your own skin and feel good about what and how you're eating.

- Happy Skinny doesn't correlate to a specific number on the scale or the size of a pair of jeans. Let's be frank: Being a size 2 isn't for everyone. Some women, such as Melissa, look and feel terrific at that size. Others, like Robin, would look bad and feel worse. Now that Robin's living on *The Skinny*, she's a size 8 (though sometimes a 6, and just once a 4). But if Robin were a size 2, she would suffer guilt and self-recrimination with every bite, and she would hardly be able to bite into a thing.

- Happy Skinny is about balancing the pleasures of eating with a sense of comfort in your body. Feeling constantly deprived because of what you're *not* eating is the road to Unhappy Skinny. Let's agree to leave that road as the one not taken.

Chapter 2

Eat What You Want

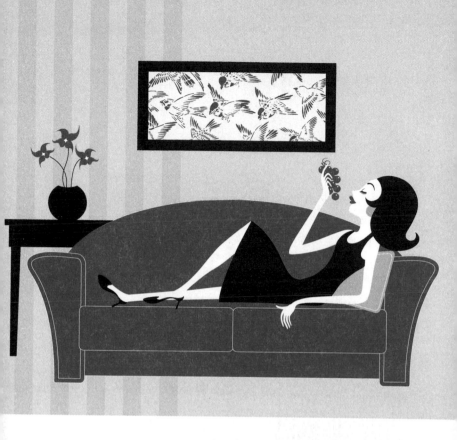

Rule #1: Eat what you want

Eat what you want. This is *The Skinny*'s number one rule. It sounds obvious, we know. But for most of us, knowing exactly what we do and don't want to eat in a given moment is not at all obvious. How many times have you stared at a menu and said, "What should I get? What are you getting? I'm just not sure." While finding your true heart's desire in work and love can be tough, when it comes to dinner, trust us, you can figure it out.

So think hard about that jelly doughnut before you pick it up. Are you going to eat it because you really want a (slightly stale) doughnut? Or do you only think you want it because it's staring up at you from the plate next to the coffee machine at work? Analyze the doughnut the same way you analyze a date: Are you going out with that nice-but-boring guy from your office because you really want to or because there's nothing new on TV?

Think some more. Instead of the doughnut, would you rather eat a handful of yummy chocolate malted milk balls, even if it means walking down to the newsstand to buy them? Would you rather go out with the guy who looks like he reads *The New Yorker* (or at least its cartoons), even if it means asking him out? Sometimes what you want most is right in front of you, but sometimes you've got to go out and rustle it up.

So before you chomp into that snackcake, or say yes to the beefcake who lives down the hall, make sure you're doing it because you really want to. When it comes to food, if you know what you really want, and get what you really want, you'll probably be happier—and skinnier—with less of it. Why? Because you're not denying yourself. You're not castigating yourself. You're recognizing your true desire in this very moment, and you're satisfying it.

Banish the guilt

You figured it out: You know what you want. You want the cookie? Have the cookie. Eating is one of life's true joys, on par with sex. And like sex, it's not about guilt and punishment. (Unless you're into that kind of thing …) Ice cream isn't a scold; it's a cold, creamy delight. Crusty white bread covered with salty butter and a slice of ham is not a mortal sin. If every time you eat, your pleasure is consumed in flames of remorse and regret, then what's the point? Lighten up. Have what you want and don't sweat it.

Oh, the pleasure, the lovely pleasure

When you eat what you want, enjoy every last bite. Swim in its sensations—the flavor, the smell, the crunch. Lick the crumbs from between your fingers. Pour them from the package onto your tongue. Appreciate the nuance in flavor and texture,

COUNT CALORIES? WE'D RATHER NOT.

We are not for counting calories because it's very hard to do accurately and it's a huge pain in the behind. But, since it came up, the average woman needs 2,000 to 2,200 calories a day to maintain her weight. You need around 1,500 calories if you don't want to be hungry all the time. Many experts recommend the 1,800 mark for losing weight, assuming you're getting moderate exercise on a regular basis (about 30 minutes a day, three to five days a week).

one (small) bite at a time. And then when it's gone, embrace its transience. Because when you're done eating, you're done. If cookies are your snack of choice and you've finished your allotment, put the bag away. Cookies are now over.

Likewise, if you want some ice cream, get an ice cream bar or give yourself a (small) scoop or two. Just Don't Eat the Pint.

And with pizza ...

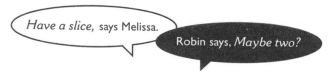

Have a slice, says Melissa.

Robin says, *Maybe two?*

but not ... you get the idea. The bottom line is this: Have a smallish portion of what's going to scratch your itch and then stop. (Stopping takes practice. See "Practice makes (mostly) perfect," page 48.)

You won't burn in hell for that cookie

You may be wondering why it's OK to eat whatever you want after reading ad nauseam in other diet books about empty calories and sugar crashes and the like. Why do we encourage you to have that cookie? To yum it up with the ice cream? There are three good reasons.

1. If you don't indulge a craving, you'll eat a million other things to substitute for the one thing you really want.

2. Once you have what you want, you can stop eating. Literally. When you really savor the food you want, the flavor will carry you, and you won't want to eat more because you will have met your emotional need for that specific food. (This is assuming you're eating reasonable and regular meals throughout the day, you're not letting yourself get superhungry, and you're not only eating processed foods that will leave you hungrier sooner.) And when you don't eat more, you eat less. Eureka!

3. No matter what anyone says, a calorie is a calorie is a calorie. To lose weight, you've got to eat fewer calories each day than you burn off. And to stay slim, you can't eat more calories than you need. So when you eat what you want and stop eating when you're done, you've probably eaten less and consumed fewer calories than you would if you substituted three different things for the one thing you wanted in the first place. See?

It boils down to this: When it comes to your waistline and that little black dress, portion size is everything. Every. Last. Little. Thing. We'll say it again and again and again. When you know what you want, you can eat what you want, but you can't always eat *all* of what you want.

Make your shoe philosophy your eating philosophy
If you wouldn't wear the same shoes every day (and who would?), why eat the same thing every day? It sets you up for boredom and bingeing. (Because when you're bored, you need

WHEN DESIRE STEERS US WRONG

Here's our one cautionary note about eating what you want: If you find that every day you want a slice of pizza and a chocolate-caramel bar or a bag of fries and three scoops of ice cream, then it's worth taking a step back and a hard look at your cravings. Fried foods and sweet foods are good to eat some of the time, but not all of the time. If you want them all of the time, then you may want to consider keeping an annotated food journal.

By writing down what you ate and how you felt when you ate it, you can start to sort through your cravings and the emotions that come along with them. We've all eaten because we're sad or lonely or pissed off or stressed out. But eating isn't the best coping method for these strong emotions. (For that matter, *not* eating isn't such a great way to cope with emotional storms either.) A journal may help you identify why you want what you want, which can be the key to knowing that you want it from a place of flavorful desire as opposed to a place of emotional dissatisfaction.

And if keeping a journal helps you recognize some big emotional trends that tag team with your food trends, we'd encourage you to talk to a professional therapist or counselor who specializes in food issues.

to break out, go wild, and throw caution to the wind with a burger! Fries! Brownie sundae! New pair of Jimmy Choos!)

So before you say you're about to eat what you want because we just said you could—and you eat that food every day so you know you want it—ask yourself, "Do I *really* want that thing I eat every day *again*?"

Don't eat the ice cream or the tuna sandwich just because that's what you always have. We know: You apply the same lip gloss in the morning and have a cookie every afternoon, a bowl of pasta every Tuesday night, and a turkey wrap most days for lunch. But that's not getting what you want—it's not even getting what you need. Unless you have a crush on your cookie seller, it's just what you do and it's probably time to do something else (and to get a new lip gloss too).

This isn't about the cookies or turkey sandwiches or plates of pasta. It's about habits, and habits are a heartbeat away from ruts. So before you eat anything one more time because it's there in front of you, stop.

Step away from the counter.

Ask yourself: "Is this what I really want? Can I get what I really want?"

Now here's the really beautiful thing. You may not be able to get those gorgeous $600 boots you spied last week. You may have to wait on the cuddly cashmere sweater. But what you really want for dinner? You can probably get that. Eat the thing you want most, and don't eat something simply because you always do.

Rule #2: Don't eat what you don't want

There you are, sitting in your pretty dress at your best friend from summer camp's wedding, when—plop!—down in front of you comes a plate of poached salmon with creamy dill sauce, julienned carrots, haricots verts, and wild rice. The salmon looks a little droopy, a little pale, a little *sad*. The vegetables look somewhat appealing (though they're likely drenched in butter and salt), while the rice looks like it's seen better weddings.

But across the table there are fresh, warm rolls with butter, and they look mighty, mighty good. Yes, the salmon is a good, healthy protein choice. It's what you're supposed to eat, but you don't want the salmon. You want a roll slathered with butter. Can you guess what we'd recommend?

You got it. Don't eat what you don't want. Instead, have the bread with a little pat of butter (the fat will help fill you up, plus it tastes great) and eat the vegetables, but skip the fish and rice (even if the rice is whole grain).

There's no reason to wade through a protein you don't like just because it's a protein, because proteins have calories just like carbs have calories. Don't eat something that you don't want when something more appealing is right in front of you.

But what if you don't have a choice? You're hungry, you're tired, you have to eat something, and it doesn't really matter what it is. We've all been there. What do you do? You eat, but don't eat everything.

THE CRASH AND BURN

Melissa can have gummy bears for breakfast and not get cranky. If Robin ate only gummy bears for breakfast, however, she'd have a stomachache and then get hungry and then turn bitchy. And she can be one hell of a bitch. It's simply not enough food for Robin, and it would lead her straight into the oft-described cycle of sugar high, sugar crash, serious hunger.

Why? For the simple reason that simple sugars in baked treats and processed sweets (such as gummy bears) have been stripped of every natural element other than their sweetness. Unlike the complex sugars (aka carbs) found in whole grains, fruits, and vegetables, simple sugars have nothing for the body to break down—no husk, no fiber—and so nothing slows down digestion. Therefore, simple sugars are rapidly absorbed by the blood, sending blood sugar levels sky-high and triggering the production of insulin in order to bring them back down. You get that lovely little buzz, but then there's nowhere to go but down and nothing left to feel but hungry.

It's like a weekend fling with your ex. At the end there's nothing to keep you going. Just the walk of shame with a bagel.

We said it once, and we'll say it again: Portion size is everything. If you don't love what you're eating (and even if you do), but you can't or won't get something else, then don't eat everything in front of you. And if you do finish what's in front of you, don't go back for seconds.

Rule #3: Build a Skinny meal

We've gone on and on about eating what you want, not eating what you don't want, and loving what you eat. But truth be told, you can't only eat what you want. You also have to eat what you need. So to satisfy your body and soul, follow these rules for making the perfect *Skinny* meal:

- Build every meal around the thing you want most.

- Add a fruit, vegetable, or both (if it's not the thing you want the most).

- Include a protein such as an egg, cheese, tofu, or turkey.

- Round it out with a complex carb like a whole grain roll, barley salad, or whole grain crackers.

(For more on fruits and veggies, protein, fats, and complex carbohydrates—otherwise known as the nutritional requirements of a meal—turn to Chapter 7, "What Every Skinny Girl Needs," page 79.)

Let's pretend that right now is lunchtime and what you really, really want for lunch is a bag of potato chips—then what you really, really don't have is a meal. Go ahead and eat some of those chips, but also add a crisp mix of greens or a juicy pear. Are you at home? Then chop up a quick and easy Granny Smith Apple Salad with Cheddar (see recipe, page 160). It will be perfect for many reasons.

- The salad will be a lovely, fresh contrast to the delectably salty taste of the potato chips.

- The fruit and/or vegetable will give you a healthy hit of vitamins and fiber.

- The salad will cleanse your palate, which will make it easier to stop eating the chips. (Because nine times out of 10, a portion of chips is actually half the bag, not the whole thing. When you're done with half, put the rest away or throw them out.)

Now it might not have occurred to you that a bag of chips and a salad of apple and cheese could actually be enough for lunch.

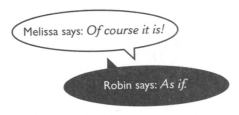

Melissa says: *Of course it is!*

Robin says: *As if.*

If that menu is just not going to cut it for you, add in more protein. Have a yogurt or whole grain bread topped with a slice of turkey breast, peanut butter, or almond butter. This will give you a reasonable variety of foods, the necessary nutrients for a meal, and those chips, your heart's true desire.

Rule #4: Don't eat to please someone else

As a food writer, Melissa eats out five nights a week, and most of the food she's served is of the heavy, just-keep-adding-butter-if-you-don't-know-what-else-to-do variety. Most of it isn't really worth finishing (granted, she's totally spoiled).

Here's her challenge: She has professional relationships with many of the chefs who feed her. And they may be insulted if she doesn't finish everything.

But Melissa won't sacrifice her waistline for someone else's feelings. Sure, if she *loves* what she's eating, and if her little black dress is sitting pretty around her belly, she may do some sauce mopping. But on a normal night, even if the food is terrific, at least half of what ends up in front of her goes uneaten (by her anyway; her date may intercede, or she may take it home).

If you're not a food writer who has a chef inspecting what's left on the plate, you shouldn't worry about hurting anyone's feelings by leaving food uneaten. This is true even if the cook is your best friend, her mom, or her new lover. Eat to please yourself, and to fit into your dress, and not for any other reason.

And when the waitperson comes over, frowns alarmingly at the unfinished bits, and asks whether you're enjoying your meal, smile sweetly and say, "Yes, thanks."

MELISSA'S DESSERT DILEMMA

Once my always-leave-food-on-the-plate habit got me into trouble. I was dining at a brand-new, superhot restaurant, and I loved the food but was self-protectively adhering to my *Skinny* policies. So I ate my usual few bites of the first four courses. As I was waiting for my fifth and final course, the waitperson nervously approached the table.

"I'm so sorry," she stammered, "but the chef won't send you dessert. He assumes if you didn't finish your meal you must not be hungry anymore."

True, I wasn't hungry anymore. But I sure as hell wanted dessert. At this fancy place, though, there was payback for not cleaning my plate.

The Takeaway

- Know what you want.
- Get what you want.
- Eat reasonable portions of what you want. When you want foods that pack a lot of calories, eat small portions. Be honest about what you're eating. Fried oyster roll? Eat half at most. A beautiful plate of sashimi? Have at it.
- Eat slowly and enjoy it. (No guilt! That's an order.)
- If it's mealtime, always include a fruit or vegetable or both.
- If you're eating to please someone else, whether a famous chef or a family member, stop.
- If you're eating to please yourself, but you're not 100 percent sure if you're pleased by the food, stop. Ask yourself if what you're experiencing while eating is really pleasure and, if it is, if you could get that pleasure from a (slightly) smaller portion.

Chapter 3

Eat When You're Hungry

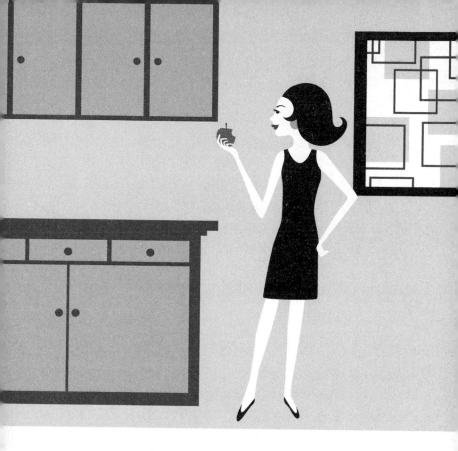

Eat when you're hungry

It's easy for us to say, "Eat only when you're hungry." But hunger isn't simple. Like sexual desire, it has many parts and involves complicated feedback loops within the body. Your brain, blood flow, hormones, senses, mood, each contributes to your ability (or inability) to recognize that you are, in fact, truly hungry and not just in the mood to chow down.

Scientists and psychologists spend a lot of time, money, and ink trying to figure hunger out in hopes that we can one day learn the secret to losing weight and keeping it off. That's all well and good, and we'll continue to read about how this hormone or that part of the brain controls the drive to eat in a way we hadn't realized before, and we'll be happier for the information. But those new insights won't change the following truths:

1. To lose weight, we must eat fewer calories than we burn in a given day. For most of us, this means eating less than we do "normally."

2. To maintain our weight, we need to eat a diet that's satisfying emotionally and nutritionally. For most of us, this means figuring out a way to balance the not-so-healthy "treats"—be they savory or sweet—with healthy, fresh foods.

So until scientists finally crack the dieting code, let's agree that in order to eat less in general—and to learn how to have our cake and eat some of it too—we've got to think a little bit about how we respond to being hungry.

How hungry? Or hungry how?

We've all experienced a variety of sensations that could be defined as "hungry." But while *hunger* is both a physiological (body) and psychological (mind) phenomenon, *eating* is primarily a behavioral one—it's all about our actions. Yes, there are hormones that send messages to our brains to tell us we need to eat. Yes, there are other hormones (leptin, for example) that let the brain know we're full. Still others (or at least one other, gherlin) tell the brain to eat more if we've stopped eating too soon.

No matter what messages our hormones send, the bottom line is the same: We must eat. But we control how, when, where, and with what we respond to our bodies' demands for food. Our responses determine how healthy we are, how slim we might get, and how sleek we might stay. Here's a look at four common ways we experience hunger—and *The Skinny* ways to respond.

Run-of-the-mill hungry

It's lunchtime, dinnertime, you-haven't-had-breakfast-yet time. You're sure you're hungry—not starving, not desperate, but also not ready to put off eating for another hour or so. Nor should you.

The Skinny response:
Use your everyday hunger to practice figuring out just what foods will give you pleasure and satisfaction.

> **Include Produce:** Whenever you sit down to eat, no matter what, include fruit and/or vegetables.

Go Fresh: Run-of-the-Mill Hungry does not warrant a king-size bag of chips or a Big Gulp, both of which are superprocessed food products. If you really, *really* want it, get it, but have just a very little bit of it—and make sure the biggest part of your meal is something fresh. The fresher the food, the better it is for you.

Remember, "fresh" doesn't mean only just-harvested, in-season foods. We're also talking a sandwich or salad or bowl of soup that doesn't come in a package and isn't full of preservatives and chemicals with names you can't pronounce.

No meal is an island: Think of your meals in relation to each other because your run-of-the-mill hunger isn't the only time you'll be hungry today. You'll need to eat again, and you probably ate already. So if you had a bagel for breakfast, eat a salad or soup instead of a panini for lunch.

HUNGER MEETS APPETITE

Hungry is *when* you want to eat; appetite is *what* you want to eat. On *The Skinny* it's important to figure out exactly what we want to eat.

If what we really want isn't around (say, smoked salmon from Russ & Daughters in New York City), then we may have to triage with what is around. But sometimes eating what you want means not eating right away (if you're not painfully hungry this is usually feasible), and waiting until something close enough to that smoked salmon becomes accessible (such as a salty Caesar salad with its anchovy tang).

It's worth waiting to eat what we want because when we eat what we want, we eat less in general, and we satisfy both our desire (aka appetite) and need (physiological hunger) quickly and completely.

I've-worked-it-baby! hungry

It's 4 p.m. on a beautiful Sunday, and you've just finished a 10-mile hike. Here you are at the end of the trail in the cute little general store, which has a few tables and an enticing menu of gourmet sandwiches and fresh soup. You know that whatever sandwich and soup you have will be oh-so-satisfying.

Or it's 2 p.m. and you're sitting down to lunch after a post-holiday sale shopping extravaganza. Even the water tastes good.

Or it's 7 a.m. and you are back from a morning bike ride. Your cheeks are flushed, your pulse is slowing, and you know that a yogurt smoothie will not disappoint.

The Skinny response:
A meal eaten to give a physically exhausted body a boost is both necessary and enjoyable. Our lives are too often too sedentary, so when we eat after physical exertion, there's a purity to it. The food tastes good and, because you're in touch with your body, you can easily tell when you're full. The experience is one in which need meets desire.

Don't overcompensate: These meals should be self-regulating. In other words, in the same way that your body tells you it needs to eat after exercise, it will tell you when it's ready to stop eating. Physical exercise usually diminishes hunger to some degree in the hours immediately following. So even if you think, "I ran five miles; I deserve to eat three slices of pizza," it's likely you and your body will actually be satisfied with one (plus a lot of salad). It's important to stay in touch with the real level of your hunger and not eat more just because you rocked out on the treadmill. That said, revel in that pizza. And have the pepperoni on top if you want it. You worked it; you deserve it.

Robin says:
Whenever I'm hungry like this—after a hike, after a long bike ride, after whatever—what I want is a sandwich.

Melissa says:
Most kinds of exercise don't make me very hungry. When I've hiked 15 miles (OK, the one time I hiked 15 miles), I subsisted on a few small handfuls of gorp, two apples, and a lot of water. I felt amazing and strong and very impressed with myself.

Robin says:

Maybe I have some weird nostalgia for hikes at summer camp where lunch was always PB&J on the mountaintop. But when I've been on my feet walking for hours, don't even think about giving me a salad. I would snarl.

Melissa says:

And all I wanted when I made it down the mountain was a hot shower, a foot rub, and a big lemonade. Shopping sales—now that gets my appetite going. And there's no better way for a girl to celebrate scoring a brand-new, pale lavender Tse cashmere V-neck at 70 percent off than a nice glass of bubbly and a plate of cured pork products.

Get-out-of-my-way hungry

This is the worst kind of hungry. You feel deprived, unnerved, angry. You ran five errands after work, and when you get home, there's nothing to eat and takeout feels like it'll take too long.

Or you're stuck in an airport after hours. All the food shops are closed and there's no hope of even a lousy sandwich on the plane.

Or you only had time for coffee at breakfast, you worked through lunch, and then you downed a handful of pretzels and some water before your 2:30 p.m. meeting. You meet a friend for dinner, and here comes the bread basket. (One word: Butter. Butter one piece of bread because the fat will help satisfy you. Eat it, then take a deep breath and pace yourself because— finally—there is a meal coming your way.)

The Skinny response:

Eating after a long, tiring day in which you didn't get enough food just isn't fun. Unlike eating after physical exertion, there's nothing exhilarating about it. It's all about getting something to eat fast and not at all about choosing or really savoring. You come to the table feeling like you've been denied and you want to make up for it. This kind of hungry is tricky because in these situations it's all too easy not just to overeat but to eat a lot of something you don't really want and then feel awful in the morning.

Slow down, part 1: Once you've secured something to eat, you must remember that it's not going anywhere. You may not have had time to eat all day, but you have time to eat now, so go slow and take a moment to focus on and really taste what you're eating. Even if you're eating a turkey sandwich and what you truly want is a rare steak, you can still enjoy the sandwich if you take a minute between frantic bites to notice that it has a yummy, salty, satisfying flavor all its own.

Slow down, part 2: By slowing down and tasting your food, you'll be less likely to eat more than you need.

Be good to yourself: At your next meal—the one after this one—treat yourself to a nice dining experience. Duck into that cute cafe on the corner for your morning coffee instead of having it at your desk. If you like to cook, take some extra time to prepare one of your favorite dishes for dinner. Have some sushi even though your budget says to have soup. In other words, remind yourself that we don't eat just to quell anxiety, and there are many, many ways to enjoy a meal.

MELISSA'S HIGH SCHOOL LESSON

When I was in high school, my health teacher, Mr. Moran, told me that the way to avoid becoming overweight was to learn how to tell your hunger from your appetite.

Hunger, he said, meant it was time for lunch. Appetite meant you were in the mood for a cookie. His advice? Don't eat that bologna sandwich in your lunch bag until you actually feel hunger pangs. These are words I still live by (sans the bologna). Now I even like it when I feel hunger pangs. They mean I've succeeded in not giving in to the first appetite-driven cookie craving that rears its furry little head. And then, well, if I feel the pangs and still want the cookie, bring it on! (After lunch, of course.)

Lay-me-down hungry (or I'm about to get my period)

We've all had these days. You wake up hungry. Not a little hungry. Exceedingly hungry. You're not sure why because you ate like a normal person yesterday. But today your hunger is not normal. You have breakfast and then you really need something just an hour later. At lunch you wolf down whatever's in front of you and wonder when you'll have your real meal. And then you go to the bathroom and, uh, Aunt Flo has come to town.

The Skinny response:
Ladies, do what you've got to do. What you do to satisfy that hunger will change as time goes on and your eating habits change. (In other words, you will satisfy even period cravings differently once you've been living on *The Skinny* for a while.) Right now? Eat what you need.

Not hungry? Feel like eating anyway?

Let's admit that for all the varieties of hungry (and we only scratched the surface) there are even more varieties of "I just want to eat." This phenomenon is most treacherous in between meals, after dinner, and on any rainy day when you're stuck at home waiting for the cable guy. In those moments or hours, your mind wanders and if your stomach grumbles just a wee little bit, you see no reason not to respond.

Here's our top 10 (actually, 11) reasons we eat when we're not hungry:

1. Boredom: Why not?

2. Stress: My boss is so working my nerves. I have to blow off steam with this bag of thick-cut kettle-cooked potato chips.

3. Deprivation: I can't have those shoes, but I can have hot cocoa with marshmallows!

4. Loneliness: Lovers come and go, but Ben & Jerry is forever.

5. Anxiety: When will I hear? When will he call? When do I get the results? Oh, forget about it, I'll have some french fries.

6. Gas: My stomach feels weird. Not bad, just weird. Wouldn't that brioche roll do the trick?

7. Easy access: There you are, cutie doughnut, sitting on that oily doily in the office kitchen just like I knew you would be.

8. Depression: This is comfort food; food is love food.

THE CALL OUT

Not eating when you're not hungry but want to eat isn't easy. You feel denied of the one thing (food) you know you can count on. So if you're struggling with saying "no" to that big serving of ice cream, enlist a friend.

- If you're at the office, instead of heading to the local Starbucks for a double macchiato with whipped cream, instant message a buddy and ask if she'll take a quick walk around the block.

- If you're home, call or email a friend.

- If no one's around or you don't feel like talking, try a new activity that will keep your hands busy: knit, needlepoint, or put together a scrapbook. Smokers do stuff like this when they're quitting, why not snackers?

9. Everyone else is doing it: Let's get nachos grande! Um, to share!

10. The holidays: See #2. Substitute Mom! Dad! Cousin Joe! You pick!

11. Reward: I made it through the morning with my preschoolers (or I finished that big project at work), and now I'm going to have my latte and scone. Just let me sit and have them all to myself.

There's no denying that food offers solace in every one of these situations. It may not be solace that actually addresses the feelings you have, but at least it's a familiar kind of comfort. We can slip into a box of Oreos just as easily as we can slip on a favorite pair of sweatpants. To make matters worse, if you're looking for a little food-love, it's for sale on every street corner in the form of a Snickers bar or bag of chicken nuggets.

Saying "no" to food when you're grumpy or moody or overextended is not simple. It takes practice. But try it the next time. See how it goes. Don't punish yourself if you have trouble abstaining; just keep trying. And then the time after that, maybe you indulge a little, but not as much as you "normally" would. And the time after that? Slowly your habits will change, and you may actually decide you don't need the comfort offered by a plate of onion rings.

Or are you thirsty?

There's one more reason we think we want to eat when we're not really hungry: We're thirsty. Despite the fact that nutritionists don't agree on exactly how much water we should drink (Eight 8-ounce glasses a day is enough! No, it's too much!), odds are that we don't drink quite enough water. So the next time you want a little taste of something, but you're not sure that you're hungry, pour yourself a low-sugar drink. (A very sweet drink will just tank up your blood sugar and make you superhungry lickety-split.) Drink some water (maybe with a spritz of lemon), seltzer (ditto the lemon), diet soda, or a big mug of tea (Robin's favorite). Often you'll find that a drink can slake your thirst and satisfy that yearning to eat.

Robin says:

So the tea trick? If you're like me and you need to have something in the midafternoon, drinking a big cup of tea is a brilliant maneuver. At least it was for me when I was trying desperately to lose any ounce of that damn last 20 pounds of baby weight. Melissa told me about this trick, and I was like, "As if." But then I tried it. And it worked! I'd make a cup of strong black tea, add a little milk and, yes, a little bit of sugar for my sweet tooth, and, really, I was satisfied. Or at least I didn't feel miserable because I wasn't eating two cookies. I'm still shocked by this.

A little hungry is A-OK

After Robin lost weight, friends asked her how she did it. She told them. They asked again. She told them again. And again. And then one day we realized they were really asking how she lost weight—or ate less—without being hungry. And you know what? She didn't. The truth is that sometimes on *The Skinny* you'll be hungry. Not painful, get-out-of-my-way hungry. But at first you may get a little hungrier before deciding to eat than you would in the past. And that's OK. Part of that hunger may come from the fact that you'll get pickier: If you can't eat something you want, you'll wait until you can. You'll begin to have a different relationship to feeling hungry, and you'll know that at some point you'll eat, and being hungry will pass.

The Takeaway

- Eat when you're hungry.
- Eat what you want, even if it means waiting longer to eat.
- If you're not hungry but want to eat, find a distraction. Call a friend, sip a cup of tea, or do some Sudoku.
- Don't use being hungry as an excuse to eat everything you can get your hands on.
- Eat fresh food. Have some grapes, a banana, or cherry tomatoes. Fruits and vegetables will satisfy your hunger at a low caloric cost.

Chapter 4

Eat Like a Food Writer

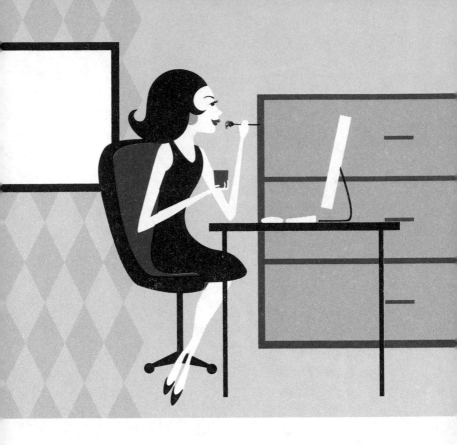

Channel your inner food writer

Here's what a food writer does whenever she finds herself close to new food: She surveys the territory. She purchases the food item that speaks to her most at that moment. Today, perhaps, it's Amish pretzel dough stuffed with mozzarella cheese and swiped with butter. She takes a few bites. She rates it by comparing it to other, related foods: "Which do I love more, pretzel sticks stuffed with mozzarella or fried mozzarella sticks? The pretzel sticks, no question." She thinks about the aroma, the texture, the flavor, and the chew. She makes a mental note to remember these for a future article. And then she throws the rest away.

Throws the rest away!?!

On the one hand, that seems wasteful, insensitive, and decadent. On the other, we are fortunate to live in a society where food is plentiful, so tossing what you don't need to eat is really a way to have just enough of what you want.

Do you need all four pretzel-mozzarella sticks? No. Do you need to eat that entire handmade, blackberry jam-filled doughnut? Unless you have your period and you Must Have Doughnut, the answer is no. Eating half will do. And let's face it, saving the second half of the doughnut for later is not reasonable because:

- It'd be messy.

- Eating the leftovers later that day would mean you've eaten a whole jam-filled doughnut, which has to be something like 2,000 calories, in one day. (And even though we don't count calories, we know that's a lot.)

- Tomorrow it will be stale and won't taste nearly half as good anyway.

So, in *The Skinny* universe, if you want your doughnut and your Isaac Mizrahi pencil skirt, toss the second half.

Toss it (no, you're not evil)

But what if your conscience won't let you toss the second half? What if you feel compelled to consume all of your completely nutritionless (if absolutely satisfying) indulgence because you spent Money and bought Food (both of which too many people don't have enough of)? You should not be a spoiled brat and throw it away. You need to finish it!

If you finish it because you *have* to, then the jelly doughnut (or ice cream sandwich or double-fudge brownie) is no longer just an indulgence. It's an indulgence wrapped in guilt and topped by punishment, and you're punishing yourself. Because if the jelly doughnut is something you crave with any regularity—and if you don't throw away at least half of your special treat—your choices turn into "No Special Treat at All" or "Gaining Weight."

Nowhere is one of your options "Eat a Whole Doughnut and Change the World." There's no practical relationship between the food on your table and the food that's not on someone else's.

If you're concerned about hunger abroad and in the United States (and we all should be), we encourage you to fight it. Volunteer at a soup kitchen or contribute to a food bank or international aid organization. Or don't eat the doughnut and instead donate that $2 to a hunger relief organization. Then you can get *Skinny* and help feed the world at the same time. But don't finish the doughnut because somewhere someone is hungry. You're not doing your waistline—or anyone else's—any favors.

Practice makes (mostly) perfect

So you're going to think and act like a food writer. You're going to get what you want, eat some of it, and throw the rest away. (And give money to a food bank or international relief organization.) Throwing away extra food involves two things:

- Determining what's extra. In other words, you must decide what your portion size will be.

- Actually stopping when you've finished your portion so that you have something left to throw away.

If you don't know how to stop eating, however, portion control is meaningless. These *Skinny* tricks can help you resist taking just one more handful of yum.

Practice in your head

Say you're at your desk and you're getting ready to have a snack. What you want is two cookies, and what you have to do is get the cookies from the platter in the office kitchen where they put the leftovers from today's meeting.

You love those cookies, and getting only two already feels like a sacrifice. So before you get up to go, take a minute. Focus on something on your desk and imagine yourself going into the kitchen, removing the plastic wrap from the tray, taking two cookies, putting the cookies on a plate, covering the tray back up, walking directly out of the kitchen, and not going back for more. Imagine yourself eating one of the cookies. And then stop.

Now, for real, get up and get two cookies. If you eat both cookies, fine. If you eat one and save one for later, fine. If you eat one and wrap one up for tomorrow, even better. If you eat one and give the second to your office mate, you've saved calories and scored niceness points. If you go back for a third cookie, don't beat yourself up about it. You can try again tomorrow. (For balancing out a splurge with the rest of your food day, turn to Chapter 11, "The Balance Beam," page 129.)

Robin says:
The first time I tried to visualize eating fewer cookies, I stood at my kitchen counter with the open cookie bag saying to myself, "Now I'm seeing myself take two cookies, take three cookies, take four cookies."

Melissa admits:
I have trouble when it comes to cookies. I love cookies above all other sweets. I especially love thick, crisp, salty, buttery shortbreads—and there's often a pan of them cooling in my kitchen. I always limit myself to two cookies. But then I always cheat by trimming shavings off the sides with a sharp knife. (This is best done while the shortbreads are still warm.) You get the idea.

Robin says: *The next time, I took three. The next, two. Now, I have no more cookies. But I will have more soon. I can see myself taking three, I mean, two …*

Melissa says: *This is not little-black-dress behavior. But it's not bad behavior either. It's just that I know if I'm going to eat 10 or so shortbread cookies, I'm sure as hell eating salad or sauteed veggies (no bread, no butter) for lunch. That's the trade-off.*

Count in your head

After you've actually eaten (not simply visualized eating, but finished chewing and swallowing), count to 100 slowly. (Count to yourself, especially if you're on a date.) This will slow down the "Yum! More!" reflex and give you time to figure out if you're sated or actually still hungry.

Whisk it away

"Take this away from me." That's what Robin's mom would say when the family was sitting around after dinner with a bag of Chips Ahoy on the table. (Hey, it was the '70s.) It's good advice.

Do not sit with open bags or big platters of food in front of you. Take what you want, then put the food away. If you can't be trusted to take the food away yourself, have someone else do it.

Leave the room

This is a bit more drastic than the "take it away" technique. You not only put the food away, you get yourself as far away from the food as possible. This is especially important when it comes to after-dinner sweets or in-front-of-the-TV snacking.

Here's what you do: After you give yourself a (smaller than usual) portion of your snack—but before you eat it—put the leftovers away. Remove your tasty treat and yourself to a whole other space, preferably on the other side of the house. It's not always easy to resist going back for more, and the closer you are to the food, the harder it is.

If you're sorely, terribly, painfully tempted to go back for seconds, try to divert yourself. Hop online, start a blog, read a graphic novel, make a collage, or give yourself a manicure.

If after all that you still go back for more, don't sweat it. Because if you start sweating the "more," you might end up throwing caution to the wind, having loads more. So keep the seconds small, enjoy them, and save the sweat for the gym.

Robin says:
I'd just given my 16-month-old daughter her first chocolate sandwich cookie. She had it in her mouth— and she started pointing to the kitchen frantically while saying, "Mo! Mo! Mo!" (That's "more, more, more" to you and me.) When I said no, she got all red in the face and started to cry and yell, "Mo! Mo! Mo!" even more insistently. She hadn't even finished the cookie and yet she was crying for more. (For the record, she didn't get it.) Isn't this how we all feel sometimes?

Throw it away, give it away

There are some delicacies so delicious that the only way to separate yourself from them is to throw or give them away. Take, for example, that rum-soaked pound cake your boss sent you for the holidays. The best, most prudent *Skinny* thing to do is to re-gift it ASAP. Wouldn't your neighbor enjoy it?

If you absolutely must have a (small) slice or two, don't put the rest away somewhere accessible, thinking you can control yourself. Admit that there's no defeating a rum-soaked pound cake. Freeze the rest immediately in one piece, wrapped in a million layers of plastic wrap. (Don't store it in the fridge in slices, which would be too easy to filch.) Better yet, give it to your sitter, your sister, or your husband to share with the office (oops, but not if it was his boss who sent it).

If that delicious something isn't appropriate to give away—say, the potato gratin in your doggy bag from last night's dinner—throw it away. Gone. In the garbage. Bye-bye. If you think it's possible that even the garbage isn't deterrent enough (and we've all been there), push the food to the bottom of the bag and take the garbage outside. Or, hell, throw some dish soap on the food.

ROBIN LOVES 'EM AND LEAVES 'EM

This room-leaving thing is exactly how my husband, David, and I manage our sweet teeth. And I have to admit it's David's control-freaky nature that got us into the habit.

We're not people who can limit ourselves to baked goods once or twice a week. No, we need them at least once a day. So after dinner (and after a piece of fruit), David puts one cookie (two if they're small) for each of us on a plate, and then we go to the family room, which is one flight up from the kitchen.

And every night I look at those two (or four) little cookies and think, "How pathetic! David's being a control freak. He's not the boss of me. Can't I have more of what I want?" And the answer is, of course, "Yes."

But I decide to wait to figure out if I want more after I've had my one cookie and started knitting. And then I think, "Is having another cookie worth putting down my knitting? I'll probably lose my place and make a mistake (because I'm a very poor knitter). Besides, I'd have to go all the way downstairs to get the other cookie, and it's so far and I'm soooo tired." Nine times out of 10, I stay put.

Become a crazy cat lady

So Melissa's go-to trick? It's called the cat-on-lap maneuver, and it only works if you have a cat and a cat-loving friend/lover/family member at hand.

Here's what you do: Sit on the couch and settle the cat snugly on your lap. Next start discussing with said friend/lover/family member the fact that a cookie would taste so good right now. But you couldn't possibly get up because the cat's pinned you down. (Note: Only true cat lovers will respond to this; everyone else will shake their heads and stare at you like you're nuts.) Sweetly ask if your F/L/FM would mind getting both of you cookies. Just one for you, please. Your F/L/FM brings you just one cookie and you eat it, and your F/L/FM eats however many cookies she wants, and the cat basks in the luxury of your lap and maybe licks the crumbs off your fingers. You can't get up to get any more cookies. And everyone is happy.

Food writers know to go slow

The hard truth is that it's hard to stop eating. We're used to eating much more food than our bodies need (our minds and souls are a different story). Once we stop eating the main part of a meal, it's tough to stop picking, especially during cleanup. (Isn't the best part of doing the holiday dishes nibbling away at the leftover crispy bits of turkey skin?)

Eating, unlike blinking or sneezing, is a voluntary behavior. Even though our bodies signal us that we're satisfied, we often don't heed that signal. Part of it is brain chemistry. Certain foods—specifically sugary ones that come at the end of the meal—turn on the brain's pleasure centers, which stoke our desire for more regardless of what our bodies need. (These are the same parts of the brain that get addicted to heroin, so don't underestimate the powerful hold a brownie can have on you.)

Another part of the problem is that we tend to eat too fast. It takes about 20 minutes for our bodies to digest our food and send the "I'm full" signal to our brains. Eating slowly and waiting between courses not only lets us enjoy our food more, it allows our bodies to recognize fullness. If we pay attention to our bodies' signals, we'll eat less overall.

So what are the food writer's tricks to knowing if she's really full?

1. Eat slowly.

2. Pay attention while you eat.

3. Listen to what your body tells you. You're probably full sooner than you think—or want to admit.

4. Practice stopping. (See "Practice Makes (Mostly) Perfect," page 48.)

The three levels of full

How does a food writer know when to say when? She follows this short guide to when enough is enough.

Full Enough

You might feel Full Enough at the end of a normal meal on a normal day when you're responding to being "Run-of-the-Mill Hungry" (page 36). Of course, "normal" is different for everyone. Melissa would feel Full Enough after eating about half of what it takes for Robin to feel Full Enough.

Don't kid yourself about how much or how little food you need. But do stop eating when you cross over the hunger line into no longer hungry. Don't think, "Am I full or not full?" Think, "Oh, I guess I'm not hungry anymore." Then stop eating. Consider these points:

- Eat what you want or something that's intensely flavored. You'll get Full Enough more quickly because the experience is more satisfying.

- Recognize that how much food you need to get Full Enough is adaptive. In other words, as you start eating smaller portions, you'll get used to it and will be sated with less food.

- Be honest with yourself about when you're Full Enough. It's often sooner than we want to admit, especially if we're eating a slice of cheesecake. But try not to feel denied or punished when you stop eating sooner than you'd like. After all, no matter how much or how little you've eaten, you'll definitely eat again in a little while (and cheesecake keeps for several days in the fridge).

Full-On Full

This is pretty darn full. You've eaten most of an appetizer, maybe a little bread, some of a main course, and some of dessert. Never mind the wine. When you get to Full-On Full you've eaten beyond your body's signals that it's Full Enough.

Full-On Full is not an everyday kind of full. It's for special dinners out (an anniversary, birthday, dinner with dear friends from out of town) or a party where the food is both delicious and lovingly prepared.

If you've been careful with your portions and you've been stopping when you're Full Enough most of the time, you'll notice you'll get to Full-On Full sooner. Once again, be honest with yourself. And stop. Or you'll land at Beyond Full (see below).

Caution: If you're out at a fancy dinner but the meal feels like a chore (perhaps you're out with clients or your boyfriend's boring cousins), resist the temptation to compensate for the tedium by eating. Because eating shouldn't be about compensating for everything your dinner companions are not.

Beyond Full (aka Unbutton-Your-Pants Full)

When you get to Beyond Full, you feel like you might not eat again for three days. This full is usually reserved for special occasions such as holiday meals with your favorite dishes that are only made once a year. Or holiday meals when you might eat a little more compulsively because your aunt or your mom is stressing you out. Or holiday meals when there's just too damn much food on the table.

Try not to reach Beyond Full more than three times a year.

The Takeaway

- Whenever you eat, eat slowly, sensuously, and completely. Then stop eating.

- Be prepared to throw food away.

- Learn what your body feels like when it's Full Enough.

- Only eat past Full Enough on special occasions.

It's All About Portions

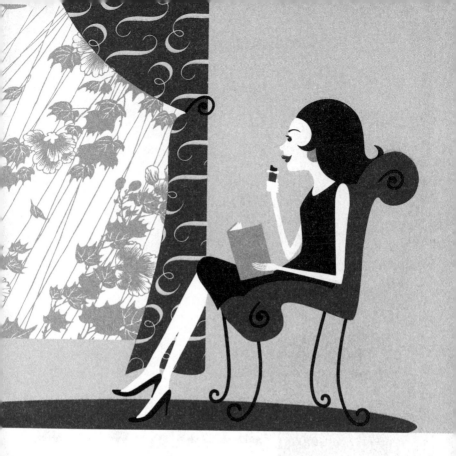

The power of portion control

Portion control is absolutely essential to living on The Skinny.

The obvious question is "What the heck is a portion?"

A portion is the amount of a certain food that you're about to eat. A portion is unregulated, except by you. You control the portion; the portion does not control you (or your pants).

A portion should not be confused with a serving, which is a technical term for a specific amount of food that's (supposed to be) standard. The FDA has serving sizes. It uses its servings to assess a particular food's calories and nutrients, which are then printed on food labels.

In *The Skinny*, we're going to refer mostly to portions because portion size is something every one of us can control.

Don't count calories

Granted, Melissa and Robin couldn't count themselves among the math geniuses in high school (or at any other time). But a fear of numbers isn't the only reason they say "No!" to the idea of counting calories.

Here's our issue with calorie counting: A calorie is a calorie is a calorie, whether it comes from a bunch of kale, a tuna sandwich, or a slice of pumpkin pie. We all know that to lose weight you must eat fewer calories than you use in a day. But calculating exactly how many calories are in everything you're eating is virtually impossible. You'd have to measure and weigh all your food and keep track of every ingredient. (How much mayonnaise is really on that deli sandwich, and does the wasabi on that spicy tuna roll add calories?) Unless you invest in an evening bag-size scale, you'd never be able to dine in restaurants. So we say, just focus on eating less (split the tuna roll with a friend and add a seaweed salad) and don't worry about the numbers.

We're not saying that you shouldn't think about how much you're eating or what you're eating for lunch in relation to what you had

THE SERVING TRAP

When you buy a bag of potato chips or a bottle of your favorite sports drink, you may think that what you're holding in your hand is one serving and that the calorie count on the back is for everything in the package. Not so fast.

Every packaged food lists the number of servings in a container. If the package you're eating contains more than one serving—and if you plan to finish the whole thing—you have to multiply the number of servings by the number of calories listed in the "nutritional content" box to calculate the number of calories you're actually eating.

Of course, we're not interested in calories (see page 26), but we're also not interested in eating the equivalent of the imagined calorie count of a triple banana split every time we open up a bag of cheddar cheese popcorn.

Bottom line: If you do want to glance at the calories on the back of the package, make sure to check out the number of servings in that package you're holding. And practice your multiplication tables.

for breakfast or will have for dinner. After all, being conscious of how much you're eating is at the heart of *The Skinny*. We are saying that it's a little exhausting to meticulously measure what you eat throughout each day. Pay attention, yes, but don't sweat the details because for the long term, you simply can't keep it up.

It's time to eat—eat a little bit less

When you sit down to eat, you need to decide how much you will eat, either by serving yourself a specific portion or figuring out when you're done with the portion given to you by, say, a restaurant or your Aunt Ida. When it comes to losing or maintaining weight, we'll say it yet again: Portion size is everything, everything, everything.

The most important thing to remember about portions is nine times out of 10, they're too big. So to keep your body feeling sleek—or to get it that way—it's worth noticing how much of the mashed potatoes you really are serving yourself.

We're not suggesting that you obsess over portions. For example, if you want to make your portion of, say, boneless chicken breast about 4 to 6 ounces, that's a piece about equivalent to the palm of your hand. But do not stand at your counter frantically comparing the breast to your hand. Instead give it a quick once over. If it looks a little big, cook the whole thing up and then cut off a piece to save for tomorrow's lunch. If the piece you cut off is small, you can throw it in a salad, have it for a snack, or feed it to your spouse or child. But don't eat it just to make your cleanup easier.

Tame the portion beast at home

When it comes to food, we've been trained to think more is more. But it's time to readjust our vision. If you're living life on *The Skinny*, what you see is what you get, and that might mean looking at less than what you're used to. Use these easy steps to help you control those portions when you're at home:

ROBIN ON LESS IS MORE

I admit it: It was hard for me to think that I could eat what looked like less food and still be satisfied. When I first started cutting back—even when I served myself what I knew to be a reasonable portion of food—I wanted to see More on my plate. Because, you know, I liked More. I had to remind myself that just because I was eating less didn't mean I would be starving five minutes after I finished. Now I can see less on a plate and know that it'll be enough (and I can have more of something else later anyway), but it took some time to get used to the more, um, "delicate" portions of food I now eat.

Measure it up

Learn how much your ladle, your big serving spoon, and any other typical serving piece you use holds by dumping the contents of said serving piece into a measuring cup. That way when you serve up a ladle full of food, you'll know what you're getting.

Next make a plate of what you consider to be an "average" serving of pasta or green beans or whatever. (Be honest about your normal serving sizes.) Measure it. Proceed to the next step.

Adjust your plate load and keep it there

Now that you know how much your serving spoons hold and what a cup of pasta looks like when it's spread out on the plate, start to scale back. If you usually cut yourself a 6-inch square of lasagna, try taking a 4-inch square. And with less lasagna taking up space on your plate, there's more room for salad or sauteed broccoli or another vegetable you love.

Repeat this step about once a month to stay on top of how big your portions are. (It's a good way to watch out for the insidious creep into bigger portions.) Once you've reached your goal weight, you can relax a little and stop measuring as often.

Split it up

Having a sandwich? Have half now and half later because you know you're going to want something later. So for lunch, have half a sandwich with some carrots, cherry tomatoes, and a big glass of sparkling water with lime. Then have the second half later in the afternoon with a nice mug of tea. (And if it's a bagel you're having for lunch? Consider making the "later" tomorrow.)

Tame the portion beast when dining out

Eat half

If it's not a humongous serving, eat a little more than half of whatever is on your plate; adjust that amount downward if the portion size is enormous. But always leave even a little food on the plate.

Split it before you get it

Let's say you're at a restaurant where you know the salad and sandwich portions are the size of your head. When you place your order, ask your waitperson to serve you half the order and pack up the other half to go. You'll probably get a funny look, but don't sweat it. It's your waistline, after all. Once home you can decide what you want to do with the other half: Save it for another meal or throw it away. Don't eat it straightaway, though. Otherwise you'd have withstood that funny look for no reason at all.

Don't order sauces or dressing on the side

After years of watching other people eat in restaurants, Melissa is convinced that when people order dressing and sauce on the side, they tend to eat more of it than they would have otherwise. So instead of getting it on the side, request that your foods be lightly dressed or sauced.

Order more appetizers and sides

Often the appetizers on a menu are more interesting than the main courses. So if you're out with someone else, order a couple of appetizers and split a main course. Or just get a couple of appetizers and a side dish, or maybe an appetizer and a side dish (and not the fried calamari and a side of garlic mashed potatoes; at least one of your choices

MELISSA'S SMALL-PLATE TRICK (IT WORKS!)

When you look at a cup of pasta spread out on your plate, does all the white space around it make you feel deprived? Then try serving your food on a smaller plate. I've used this trick ever since I realized how pathetic my usual half cup of Grape Nuts looks at the bottom of a regular cereal bowl. Intellectually, I know a half cup of Grape Nuts (mixed with a little yogurt, drizzled with honey, and topped with raspberries) will be enough for breakfast, but it still looks, well, small and wrong. The answer? I now eat breakfast out of a tea cup. It's the same amount of food, but it feels like more.

should be a salad or a vegetable dish). It may seem more like eating tapas, but you'll get plenty of food.

Honesty is the Skinniest policy

Whether you're eating at home or in a restaurant, be honest about how much you need to eat to be Full Enough (see page 53). And remember, when it comes to controlling portion size, it's all about practice. You're not bad if you eat more than what you think is a *Skinny* portion. And you're not good if you eat less. If you eat too little, you may be absolutely miserable the rest of the day and you could overcompensate by bingeing at snacktime or having a too big portion at your next meal. (Robin knows this trap intimately.)

From a practical perspective, this seesaw of too much/too little is why measuring is so handy. When you measure out, say, one cup of mushroom barley soup, you can be sure you're not getting the chintziest portion ever.

From an emotional perspective, it's useful to keep in mind that giving yourself a portion is something you practice each time. There's no absolute perfect portion and no absolute best way to eat. There's just you making your way through your day.

Melissa insists:
Two spoonfuls of ice cream eaten at your freezer have fewer calories than two spoonfuls eaten elsewhere because you're standing up.

Robin counters:
Hooey. If I stand at my freezer, I eat way more than two spoonfuls of ice cream! Give me a little bowl with two, OK, four spoonfuls, a spoon, and a couch, and I'm happy.

Less isn't more, but it's probably enough

Here's the thing: If you like to eat larger portions but you also want to lose weight and keep it off, you not only have to start eating smaller portions, you also have to accept five new realities.

1. You will finish eating before your dinner companion. There's no way around it. Even if you eat slowly (which we all should), when you're eating less, you will be lingering over your not-quite-empty plate longer. And if you're in a restaurant, lingering means picking at what's left on that plate. So talk with your hands or, you know, sit on them. Or ask the server to take your plate away when you're finished eating, even if your companion is still going (something they may not do in a fancy restaurant unless you specifically ask).

2. Even though you've eaten less for lunch, you can't eat more for dinner. This is not easy. If you're like Robin, when you eat less at lunch, you think, "I ate so little at lunch, I can eat more for my snack." Sorry. No go.

3. You can always eat more veggies or fruit if you don't feel like you've eaten enough of other foods. They're healthy and they'll fill you up (and you won't feel deprived).

4. As we've said before, if you really like what you eat, you don't have to have the biggest portion of it imaginable. If you pay attention (really pay attention) and enjoy your food the whole time you're eating, you really will be satisfied more quickly.

5. Smaller portions do not mean less enjoyment. If anything, they can bring more pleasure because you end up eating a wider variety of foods.

Here's the best news: We know from personal experience that when you start eating smaller portions, you get used to them. You get used to seeing a certain amount of food and associating that amount with "enough," and you stop thinking you can (or must) compensate for eating less the next time you head to the kitchen. It takes a little time, for sure, but it happens.

The Takeaway

- Be attentive to your portions. Don't make them too small or too big.

- When you're getting started on *The Skinny*, measure the food you serve yourself.

- Look at your (smaller) serving and think to yourself: This is enough! (And remember that you can always serve yourself a huge pile of greens.)

- If you think you've eaten too much, don't feel guilty. There's always your next meal to practice smaller portions.

- Enjoy everything you eat!

Chapter 6

Zen and the Art of the Meal

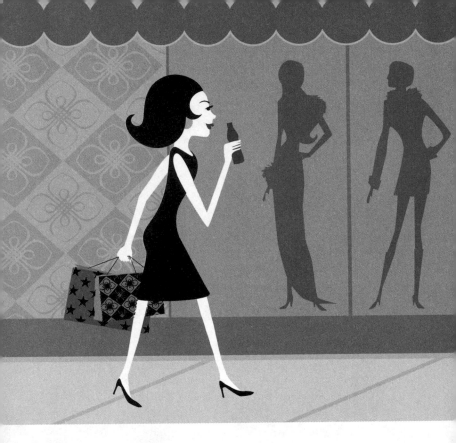

How to eat like you shop

Let's say you're about to buy a pair of boots. Not just any
boots, a pair of completely amazing Sigerson Morrison boots
that you figure are more important than this month's rent.
You see those boots across the store. You try to look away.
You walk over and pick one up. You feel the buttery suede and
admire its perfect contours. You don't even look at the price
because you know, you just know. You ask for your size. Once
they're on, you see how these boots would transform your
entire wardrobe into the realm of fabulousness.

You can't imagine living without them. So you buy them. You
convince yourself that you're actually saving money because you
won't have to buy another piece of clothing or another accessory
all year. Then you take pleasure in figuring out when you'll wear
them first. Where you'll go, what you'll do, and, of course, how
completely and utterly divine you'll look.

What does the experience of falling truly, deeply, profoundly in love with a pair of boots have to do with *The Skinny* philosophy? A lot.

Let's go back to the moment when you first met the Sigerson boots. Here's what you wouldn't do: You wouldn't grab one, hold it up for two seconds, plunk down your credit card, and then run out of the store without even noticing how they felt or looked. Would you?

And yet, how many times have you done that with a cookie? A panini? A chocolate peanut butter cup? You see it, you have to have it, you can imagine how it would taste and feel in your mouth right now. You stand there waiting for the cashier to just hurry up already. You can barely take the delay, and you eat it immediately—walking down the street. You eat it so fast that even though you know you tasted it, you can't really remember that sensation even a minute later.

This is not embracing the pleasures of the table; you're not even at a table. This kind of reaction has nothing to do with relishing your food. It has nothing to do with Happy Skinny. This, friends, is yet one more run down the road to Unhappy Unskinny.

Stop! Don't eat on the go

Why can't you remember what that thing you ate while charging down the street tasted like? Because when you eat on the run, food is just something in your mouth.

You can't experience the flavor fully because you're not paying attention. And because you're not paying attention to what you're eating, you're really not paying attention to how much you're eating.

When you eat on the run, you eat too fast and too much. And typically the food that's best for eating on the run—food you can hold in your hand—is highly processed. (Face it: You've probably never had a salad while running through an airport.)

Plus, chances are if you've ever eaten on the run, you know that you're often hungry again as soon as you get where you're going. That's because you weren't truly satisfied by what you ate while running. Your hunger might have been calmed, but your appetite—the part of hunger that wants to enjoy specific foods—is hanging on, demanding its turn at the banquet.

So, you know what? Skip this whole fiasco. Run on the run, don't eat on it. Instead, wait until you have a moment to sit and enjoy your turkey wrap or your banana. It's worth waiting for.

> **Melissa says:**
> *Speaking of running. We don't mean to nag, but how's that exercise thing going?*

Skinny girls eat on the slow

If you're living life on *The Skinny*, you only eat standing still or, better yet, sitting still. (And not while driving your car.) You look at what you're eating, inhale deeply, and savor the smell of the food. (Melissa always smells something before she eats it; it's a must-do for food writers to get the full sensory experience.) You always take a moment before you dive in to really appreciate what's in front of you and let a little anticipation build.

Think of it as foreplay for your meal. It adds to the pleasure. If you have to eat fast or while traveling (that is, on the run), give yourself five minutes to devote to making your quickie a nice experience (and there's nothing wrong with the occasional quickie). Chew your food completely and sip, don't gulp, your water (or iced tea or whatever).

We know it doesn't always feel like you have even five minutes to spare. Life is busy. We have a lot to do: Too many errands, too many hours at work, too many phone calls to return, and too many plans for organizing our closets to ponder. But none of that changes the basic fact that we must eat, and if we eat an average of five times a day (three meals, two snacks), we should try to give our bodies and our food the respect they deserve by eating every meal with some care and attention.

In other words, treat your food like a new pair of $600 Sigerson Morrison boots, or at least like a $150 (on sale) pair of slides. Make eating an experience you enjoy. And you can do that in five minutes, 20 minutes, or three hours.

If you don't have five minutes to spare for eating? Don't eat. Have a big bottle of water or a milky tea or coffee and just wait until you can take the time (even if it is just a few minutes) to enjoy your food. Chances are your hunger will mellow in a few minutes anyway; it usually does unless you're truly underfed.

EATING ON THE FLY

Airplane food is, by and large, not good. So *The Skinny* girl brings her own meals with her on airplane trips. Use these tricks for eating well on the fly:

- Crisp veggies hold up well for several hours without refrigeration and can be packed in spacesaving plastic bags. Try steamed or roasted green beans, asparagus, broccoli, and cauliflower; raw carrot and celery sticks; peeled whole Kirby cucumbers; sliced red bell peppers; and heads of endive, which peel apart and taste great paired with cheese.

- Choose less-juicy fruits such as apples and Bosc pears; they're easier to eat on a plane than, say, peaches. Or go for dried fruit.

- Avoid bananas unless you plan to eat them in the airport. They always get smooshed.

- Pack grapes and cherry tomatoes in sturdy plastic containers.

- Avoid really stinky cheeses as a courtesy to your fellow passengers. Good choices include hard cheeses such as aged cheddar, Manchego, Parmesan, pecorino, or Stilton. These tend to stink less than soft, strong ones.

- Whole grain crackers hold up better than bread; soft bread tends to get squashed, and crusty bread is really messy to eat.

- Hard salamis and sausages are terrific. Cut them into chunks ahead of time; chunks won't stick together like slices can.

- If you want to pack sandwiches, cut them into small pieces and wrap them separately before you leave the house. Cramped quarters can make eating a hero a hazard.

- A cookie or two, or a few squares of chocolate, is nice.

- Pack a few prepackaged wet napkins, just in case.

Robin says:

Melissa makes all the meals she serves to friends pretty and special in some way. So I assume she makes all her own meals pretty. Except the ones she claims to eat over the sink. Stop that, Mel!

Melissa says:

Robin's right. (And I'm working on that sink thing.) Whenever I have friends over to dinner, I try to make it special, even if it's just two of us ordering in on a weeknight. I light a few candles, use cloth napkins, and set out nice wineglasses, whether we're sipping wine or seltzer. It elevates even steamed shrimp and vegetables to company-food status.

Set the stage (then clean it up)

Visual cues are an important part of our lives. We put familiar objects on our desks or take a treasured photo with us when we travel. The things we see settle us. So while you're getting used to life on *The Skinny*, set up an attractive visual space for your meal or snack.

If you're at your desk, clear a space and use a napkin as a place mat. If you're home alone, put the food on a plate, dress your table (it can be your coffee table), and pour yourself a glass of wine if you like. And when you're done with your meals, put things away, signaling to yourself that you're done eating. The meal is now over. You will eat no more for now.

Say no to mindless munching

Eating on the run isn't the only time we eat too much too quickly, without thought. We do it often and everywhere—at desks, on couches, in hallways, standing over the kitchen sink. Wouldn't it be great if we had sex in all the places we overeat? (By the way, when you kiss for 30 seconds you burn 30 calories. Not that we're counting calories …)

The point is to banish the hallmarks of mindless munching from the majority of your encounters with food. You're guilty if you:

- Choose to eat whatever and not what you really want

- Eat without putting your food down

- Eat without looking at your food

- Eat without tasting your food

- Eat without breathing

- Eat without noticing how much you've eaten until it's nearly or all gone

It's not so easy to stop eating like this because foods are made and packaged to be "convenient." They're in "snackable" sizes, so often you don't have to think about portion size. But eating without thinking is eating without joy.

Yet every time you sit down zombielike in front of the television with a bowl of microwave popcorn and finish the whole thing, you're reinforcing the idea that mindless eating is relaxing and pleasurable.

But is it?

Well, sort of. We admit there's something pleasurable about mindless eating, but it isn't about food. The pleasure of food

THE PLEASURE OF FOOD PREPARATION

Here's what's nice about making your own food: You get to make it. Even if you're simply peeling an orange and sprinkling it with olive oil, salt, and a fresh herb or two, you're making something that wasn't there before.

The process is fun and satisfying. Even when we're bone tired and couldn't care less about slicing an onion, doing so can be creative, reassuring, and rejuvenating. That's not just because we like food but also because cooking allows us to make some kind of small connection with the meal we're about to eat.

Cooking also makes the start of a meal easy to notice: The meal starts when you start preparing it. Your anticipation builds as you add a dash of pepper here, a sprig of rosemary there. Preparing fresh food—even if "cooking" means drizzling some homemade dressing over bagged baby spinach—doesn't have to take a lot of time, but it is time well spent. Fresh food, made by you, satisfies your hunger and your soul.

comes from its flavor and texture and smell, and you're not noticing these things if you're paying attention to the TV.

MELISSA'S MEAL CHECKLIST

Here's what I believe every *Skinny* gal needs to set the visual stage for a meal:

• A napkin or three (one for your place mat, one for your lap, one for cleanup)

• Real cutlery, including a knife, fork, spoon, and serving spoon

• A glass for what you'll imbibe

• A designated eating area, even if it's just your lap

• Candles, flowers, and nice music. These are strictly optional but will definitely improve your experience (though you might get funny looks if you try this at work).

The pleasure in mindless munching stems from just being mindless. There's a kind of relief in not thinking, especially when the rest of your day is spent trying to finish one thing while getting a head start on that other thing and running to this and making sure you did that. When you finally sit down in front of the flickering TV with that popcorn—and you don't have to do a thing other than bring hand to mouth, over and over again—it can feel like a great relief.

And that's fine. But what it won't do is give you the true pleasure of what you're eating. And life on *The Skinny* is about a life rich in pleasure. Food is too wonderful, and our bodies too important, to squander the joys of eating so carelessly. Apply the pleasure principle wherever you are, not just in front of the TV.

Be present in the moment

Eating should be a sensual experience, so when you stop noticing what your food tastes like, you should stop eating. That sounds logical, right? Let's say you're eating a big, warm, fudgy brownie topped with scrumptious vanilla ice cream. The first few bites taste great. You're loving the way the melty-gooey chocolate makes yum-puddles with the sweet cream.

There is no obvious moment when a bell goes off and you say, "The pleasure is done." But there will be a moment when the novelty will wear off. When the shocking jolt of cold vanilla mixed with a warm bed of intense chocolate stops being quite so shocking. When you know what you'll taste when you next bring the spoon to your mouth. When the top of your mouth goes the slightest bit numb from the chill and you stop distinguishing the brownie from the ice cream and start experiencing something that's mostly sweet, cold, and chewy.

That's when you stop. (This is probably about a third of the way in.) You might not want to stop, but you can and should because if you stop at this point you still have had a fully satisfactory encounter with a sweet sensation. And if you want to lose weight or keep it off, really, it's time to stop.

Remember too: You will have that food delight again, some other time. And that's why you don't need so much of it right now. The pleasure of the decadent dessert is not gone from your life; it's just intensified into a more condensed, but ever-so-satisfying encounter.

AN EATING MEDITATION

We first read about this eating technique in Jon Kabat-Zinn's classic book, *Full Catastrophe Living*. It will help you learn how to savor every element of a meal. So, with a thank you (again and again) to Dr. Kabat-Zinn, here goes:

Take three raisins (or grapes or peanuts or dried apricots) and lay them in front of you. Look at each raisin. Pick one up, look at it, feel it in your hand, notice where your arm is, your hand, as it holds the raisin. Smell it. What associations does the raisin trigger? Do you even like raisins? Slowly and carefully, noting the movement in your arm, back, and head, bring the raisin to your mouth. Are you salivating? Eat the raisin. Chew it thoroughly and feel it rolling around in your mouth. What happened to the hand that was holding the raisin? Where is it?

Repeat this with the second raisin and then the third, noting how you feel at each stage and with each raisin.

Imagine, just imagine, bringing even a fifth of this attention to a regular meal. How much more would you taste? Experience? Feel? And dare we say, how much more quickly would you recognize that you have been satisfied by your food and can stop eating?

Food ruts: Cousin of the mindless munch

What's so bad about eating the same chicken salad sandwich for lunch every single day? If you weren't reading this book in hope of changing your lifestyle and eating habits so that you'll fit back into that little black dress, we'd say, "Nothing at all."

But the fact is, if you're stuck in a food rut, it's worth looking at and trying to change.

Food ruts are easy to fall into because of three things: access, ease, and comfort. We know certain foods, they reassure us, they're easy to make or get, and they're nearby. And let's face it, when you go food shopping it's tough to stop buying the same stuff and start buying something new because it would mean planning, reading a recipe, writing down the new ingredients, and all that. And all that takes time and energy.

But breaking out of your food rut will reward you with more varied, interesting meals and snacks. Those new flavors mean you're likely to be more quickly satisfied (because you pay more attention to what's new than to what's comfortable), and that will probably make it easier for you to eat less of the new thing, no matter how tasty.

We know this sounds counterintuitive. Like, "What? I'm going to make a new food that I think is delicious and then eat less of it than I would of an old food that I eat all the time?" But trust us on this one. It's all about the attention you bring to the new food. New food demands more attention. A more varied diet means a more interesting diet, and a more interesting diet will keep you from falling into the mindless monotony of the same old thing and remind you how compelling new foods in small(ish) portions can be.

This said, if your food rut consists of eating a cup of cherry tomatoes every day at 4 p.m. as a snack, or it means drinking the same fat-free soymilk banana-berry smoothie every day for breakfast—and if it makes you happy to have that healthy routine—feel free to stick with it. Everyone else, read on.

Breaking a food rut at home

1. Every other time you go to the market, get something you haven't made at home before or in a long while. Rice noodles, watercress, mangoes for mango avocado salsa, whatever.

> **Robin says:**
> When it comes to new foods, Melissa is my inspiration. She eats and makes new things all the time. Sometimes I get kind of bummed when I eat at her house because if I really love something, I know I'll never have it again; she hardly ever makes anything twice. (Except on her birthday when she always serves bagels and lox.) I firmly believe that because she's always trying a little bit of something new, she is always engaging her taste buds. This is not to say there are no familiar comfort foods at Chez Melissa. (One word: shortbread.) But it is to say that because she eats so many different things, she avoids the traps of complacency, which are (1) eating a lot of food that you (2) don't taste much because you eat them so often.

2. Buy a new food magazine or search a new food website to get new recipe ideas. Then make one new dinner recipe at least every other week.

3. Ask your office mate, your hairdresser, and your neighbor what they like to make for dinner and use that to spark ideas.

4. Create variations on your favorite recipes. If you always make baked salmon, try substituting tuna or red snapper. Bored with your usual beef meat loaf? Use ground turkey or veal or pork. And if you can't bear to look at another chicken breast, cook turkey or tofu using the same seasonings.

5. Look in your pantry. If you have more than three cans of chickpeas and four boxes of your kids' favorite cracker, it's time to find some new legumes and crackers.

Breaking a food rut away from home

A food rut when you work outside your house is different from a food rut when you work in your house. The out-of-the-house food rut involves routines such as where you go for your morning coffee, the three convenient places you head for a snack, and the people you always go to lunch with.

It's hard to break these ruts because when we're tired and stressed and harried and late, we depend on our routines to help things run smoothly. But if your day is going pretty smoothly, and you're not craving the tomato-dill soup from the place where you always get tomato-dill soup, try something new.

Of course, you may not think you're in a rut at all. But if you've had turkey sandwiches more times than you can remember in the last two weeks, or if you've had strawberry yogurt at 10 a.m. every day for as long as you've been at your job, you're in rut city.

Try these ideas to break out of your routine:

1. Order something you've never had before, even if you're at the same place you always go.

2. Try a new place.

3. Make something new and bring it in for breakfast or lunch (see recipe section, page 141).

4. Take a different route to work, one that doesn't involve passing by the doughnut shop.

IS IT A RUT?

If you're not sure how often you eat the same five things, keep a food journal for two weeks. If you can write "ditto" three or more lunches in a row, you're in a rut. By forcing you to pay closer attention to your food, a journal will help you identify your strongest habits and the food areas that need the biggest shape up. Keeping a journal is a big commitment. While we don't think it's a habit that's sustainable (and we're all about cultivating attitudes that are sustainable long term), it can be helpful.

5. If there's a candy jar on your desk, get rid of it; make sure the bowl is opaque (you'll eat less if you can't see it, according to one study) or fill it with candy you don't really like.

6. Take a walk instead of eating a snack (but don't walk near that doughnut shop).

7. Shake up your beauty routine: Buy new lipstick, wear your hair up, get new earrings.

From Robin:

I confess that I'm in a snack rut. In the afternoons I love to eat two squares of very dark chocolate and a small handful of almonds. Now the thing is, when I started this chocolate habit, I ate more than two squares and then, seriously, I'd get a stomachache. I know that sounds very Princess and the Pea-ish, but more chocolate (at one sitting) made me, uh, peevish. But those two squares? Stand back. I have to have them.

Melissa says:

I go through snack ruts that last for a few weeks at a time. For a while it was a slice of avocado sprinkled with sea salt on rye crisp crackers. Then I moved on to a square of cheddar eaten with very sour gherkin pickles. Now I'm in my cut-up-apple-spread-with-a-little-almond-butter phase. Who knows what will come next?

The coworker rut

Work friends are a special kind of friend. We spend a lot of hours with this group of people whom we haven't always chosen, and when you find someone or a few people you really like at work, those relationships become hugely important. They help you manage the stress of your job, no matter how much you love what you do.

It's natural that because eating is one thing we all have in common, food can play a big role in the workplace—talking about it, sharing it, getting it for free (leftover croissants from the breakfast meeting). Mealtime is like recess, and nobody likes a spoilsport.

So you may be worried about what your coworkers will think if you suddenly say no to the Tootsie Rolls in the candy bowl. And if you all lunch or snack together regularly, you might not want to draw attention to yourself or your new habit of eating an apple instead of the usual cookie or ordering a salad instead of a meatball hero.

The thing is, just because they're your friends doesn't mean you have to tell them everything about what you're eating and why, and you certainly don't have to eat for their benefit or to stave off questions about why you're not having your fair share from the fried chicken bucket.

Sharing a meal or even a snack with someone is about companionship. If eating with a certain someone starts to feel like it's competitive or like you're being judged, do not eat with that person. Who needs that? Have coffee, have tea, but do not have a meal.

The Takeaway

- Do not eat on the run.
- Do not eat like you're on the run when you're on your couch.
- Do not confuse mindless munching with pleasure.
- Set your table as often as you can.
- Avoid food ruts.
- Cook using fresh food as often as you can.
- Truly, deeply, and madly enjoy your food as often as you can.

Chapter 7

What Every Skinny Girl Needs

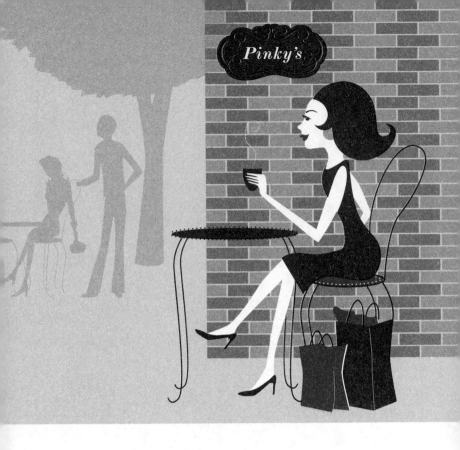

It's fruits and veggies

A long time ago, many years before the creation of *The Skinny*, there was just Melissa, preaching dieting advice to all who asked the question: "How can you be a food writer and stay so slim?"

Back then, before she actually sat down and analyzed the behaviors and strategies that went into maintaining her waistline (and are set down in this book), her answer was simple: "Eat more fruits and vegetables."

Of all the tricks she used to stay svelte, eating more fruits and vegetables was the cornerstone, the golden rule. That's because not only are they good for your health, but they fill you up, so you will probably eat less of everything else.

Give them a try. Once you start eating more fruits and veggies, it becomes second nature. Roasted chicken will start to look sad without mounds of green salad on the side, and your afternoon snack won't seem complete without a handful of baby carrots.

The world of produce is vast, exciting, and extremely tasty, if you know how to prepare it. (Need a jump-start? Check out our recipe section, page 141.) We say, dig in.

The Skinny on vegetables

Do we really need to tell you this again? OK. Eat vegetables. Eat carrots, artichokes, asparagus, bell peppers, mushrooms, eggplant, and greens (mustard, kale, broccoli rabe). The list could go on and on. Vegetables have vitamins, minerals, antioxidants, phytonutrients (plant-based nutrients), and fiber. They contain a lot of water, so they'll make you feel full. Make them the base of your meals and garnish them with proteins. You simply can't go wrong with a vegetable-rich eating routine.

All *The Skinny* recipes (see page 141) are based on the premise that if you eat more veggies (and fruit, of course) with smaller but still substantial portions of protein (about 6 ounces of meat, chicken, tofu, fish, eggs, or cheese), you will lose weight and/or keep it off.

Use veggies to satisfy your hunger. Fill up on them before you dive into that ooey-gooey-decadent treat. Want a root beer float for dinner? Have a pile of sauteed broccoli rabe first. How about that burger with a fried egg on top? Swap out the fries for a salad or sauteed spinach. Need the fried calamari? Add a fennel-and-orange salad or a big bowl of vegetable soup to it. The bottom line? Vegetables are your friends—get to know them better.

THE ONE-NIGHT VEGGIE

Not every vegetable is your long-term, tried-and-true friend. Some vegetables are more about a slightly drunken one-night stand. (You should only have them every so often.) Steamed broccoli? Best friend forever. Broccoli with cheddar cheese sauce? A roll in the hay. Moroccan Carrot Salad with Coriander and Cashews (page 172)? Bring it home to mama. Maple-glazed carrots? Just take 'em once around the block.

Of course a dish like maple-glazed carrots is often served alongside something even more decadent like macaroni and cheese. In this case, choose the lesser of two evils. (Yes, it's the maple-glazed carrots.) Whenever faced with vegetables fancied up with heavy cream sauces and sweet glazes, eat them strategically.

Starchy versus nonstarchy veggies

Starchy vegetables naturally contain a lot of sugar, so they should be treated like grains in your diet: Eat them, enjoy them, and savor them, but don't use them as the basis of your diet like you would nonstarchy vegetables. Common starchy veggies include corn, potatoes (white and sweet), pumpkins, winter squashes (butternut, acorn, pumpkin), peas, and parsnips.

Beans, seeds, and nuts

Beans, seeds, and nuts—also called legumes—come from plants that bear seeds we can eat. Legumes include beans (black-eyed peas, chickpeas, kidney beans, black beans, white beans), lentils, split peas, soybeans, and peanuts. On the one hand, legumes are starchy. But they also have protein, almost no fat, absolutely no cholesterol, and folate, potassium, iron, and magnesium. And they are filling. And they are very good for you. So, you know, eat them.

The Skinny on fruit

We know you have a friend who did it. She went on some no-carb diet and—because fruits have carbs (aka sugar)—spent two weeks fruit-free. News flash: Forget about the carb-free craze. It's so over. It's time to embrace your inner Eve and eat all the fresh fruit you can get your hands on. Don't sweat the sugar in fruit and do not limit yourself when eating it. Fruit is delicious and healthful, full of vitamins and minerals. If you're craving something sweet, it will satisfy you. More to the point, a piece of

FIBER-LICIOUS

Fruits, vegetables, and legumes are fiber-filled foods. More specifically, they're full of insoluble fiber. Not only can't insoluble fiber be digested, it slows down digestion, which means the energy from fiber-rich food is released more slowly so you feel satisfied longer.

Grains and oats also contain fiber, but it's soluble fiber. It does good things too, like lower your bad cholesterol and blood sugar level.

So feel good about the fiber. When you eat a lot of both kinds, you'll lower your risk for heart disease, diabetes, and ailments of the digestive tract. You'll also be full and "regular" (you know what we mean).

fruit has a lot of water and a lot of fiber, and both will fill you up with a minimal amount of calories. So eat more fruit.

> Melissa says:
> *A banana is your friend. Enjoy one today—plain, in a smoothie, with some cottage cheese. It's filling, full of potassium, and tasty. Ignore any carb-phobic bad banana press.*

A gal can't live on fruit alone

Fruit alone often makes the perfect snack, but sometimes it's not enough to keep you full as a meal. If you find this to be true, add a protein and/or a good fat. For example, have fruit with yogurt or cottage cheese for breakfast, or fruit and oatmeal made with milk. For a snack, have the classic fruit-cheese combo (apple and sharp cheddar or good Parmesan, pear and blue cheese, grapes and goat cheese). Or have an apple smeared with peanut butter or almond butter (no more than 1 tablespoon; measure it and you'll see it's actually a lot). The combination of protein, fat, fiber, and water will help you get and stay full, and the intense flavors will leave you happy and sated.

MAKE IT OBVIOUS

Here's the thing: If you have fruit around, you'll eat it. Keep some oranges or apples or mangoes on your table and you'll be more likely to have a piece after dinner. Keep a kiwi or two on your desk and you'll find that it makes a good snack (just cut the kiwi in half and scoop out the flesh with a spoon). After you buy that fruit (melon, pears, whatever), cut it up and put it in a plastic container in the fridge so it'll be easy to grab. Fruit isn't "just like candy," but just like candy, if you keep it close, you'll reach for it.

The dried and the juiced

Steer clear of fruit juice. Fruit juice has all the sugar and all the calories of a piece of fruit but without the fiber. In essence, having fruit juice is like having a candy bar or a soda pop. If you're susceptible to a sugar rush and crash, fruit juice will set you on that course.

Dried fruit (apricot, fig, date) retains the fiber and sugar of fresh fruit but loses most other nutritional value. A piece or two of dried fruit can be a sweet, chewy snack that's as yummy as a cookie and at least gives you fiber to fill you up. But in general, eat dried fruit sparingly. Use it as a complement to, say, a small handful of nuts. Mixing a scant few raisins in with your peanuts makes them taste as good and sweet as honey-roasted nuts and is slightly more nutritious and less caloric to boot.

> Robin says:
> *When I was pregnant, I ate nonstop. My husband said I was like an eating machine. I couldn't help it. I was really, really hungry! And I ate like this a lot: apples and peanut butter, apples or pears and cheese, cottage cheese and bananas, yogurt and berries and bananas. I always had a protein with my fruit, and it always soothed my hunger, which was no small feat.*

The Skinny on buying produce

If you're not used to buying a lot of fruits and vegetables, and even if you are, here are some things to consider:

1. **Make 'em fresh.** In other words, buy your fruit in the produce section of your supermarket or at the farmer's market as often as possible.

2. **In season is good.** Why? In-season fruits and vegetables taste better. If you don't believe us, do a side-by-side taste test this August of a tomato from your neighbor's garden (or a farmer's market) and a "hot house" tomato from your local Super-Duper market. The hot house tomato? Edible. Your neighbor's tomato? Nectar from the gods.

3. **Local is good.** Why? Because if it's local, that apple didn't have to travel across the country or halfway around the world to get to your table. If it's local, it's

probably from a smaller farm. Smaller farms tend to use growing methods that are more environmentally sustainable than those used by big, profit-hungry agribusiness farms. By sustainable we mean methods that will not wrench every last bit of goodness from the ground while burying boatloads of chemicals in it—all for more profits. We mean methods that help the land regenerate. And we mean methods that cannot use the economies of scale that big agribusiness uses.

You might not be able to buy all of your fruits and vegetables from local farmers. In the winter you might want to eat something other than root vegetables if you live in a cold climate. But if you can make room in your food budget for the local stuff—even just one bunch of spinach or a bag of apples—then even that much is good for you and the earth.

4. **Find a farmer's market.** These markets are fantastic sources for local fruits and vegetables. Not only is the produce as fresh as can be (much of it was picked early that morning), there's also a richer, more interesting selection than at the supermarket. And because the produce is fresher at farmers' markets, it will keep longer once you get it home. To find a farmer's market near you, go to the USDA's website at www.ams.usda.gov/farmersmarkets/map.htm.

5. **Choose organic or close to it.** Organic fruits and vegetables carry a lighter pesticide load or none at all. This is very important for kids because "safe" levels of pesticides are determined based on the weight and metabolism of an adult, not a child. But even for adults, it's a safe bet that organic foods introduce fewer toxins into your body. Plus by buying organic foods, you're supporting farming that uses fewer chemicals and so is better for you and better for the earth. Getting "organic" certification from the government requires jumping through many, many hoops. Not every small farm has

the time or money to do it. If you're at a farmer's market, ask the farmer at the stand if he or she uses pesticides. Some farmers might not be certified organic but still grow their food with minimal pesticides.

6. **Use the freezer strategically.** Frozen fruits and vegetables are useful, and even if some studies suggest they're not quite as nutritious as the fresh, they're better than nothing. You can even buy organic frozen vegetables and fruits. Robin gives her kids organic frozen vegetables, which are convenient because she can cook up a serving size right before lunch or dinner and not worry about how quickly the rest is going bad. We both use frozen berries during the winter to make smoothies.

7. **Avoid cans.** Canned fruits tend to come packed in heavy, sugary syrup that adds many unnecessary calories. Canned vegetables tend to be highly salted.

SHOULD YOU BAG THE BAG?

There are all kinds of prepackaged fresh produce products—such as spinach, lettuce, baby carrots, and sliced apples—available at your local supermarket. They're great because they make food preparation easy, easy, easy. Who doesn't love easy?

But even though the package might say "prewashed," you should wash that produce anyway. Some consumers have found themselves sick, at times seriously, from food-borne bacteria present in bagged produce. Bacteria are a problem with these products because the supply chain, or the system that gets the produce from the fields to market, is long. Many people come in contact with the products, and the production and handling processes aren't regulated.

Voluntary regulations have been established, but you can't always be sure they're being followed. But don't bag the bags if it means eating less produce. Instead, just give that produce a good rinse.

Melissa says:

I often buy prepackaged fruits and vegetables, but I do have one bugaboo: spring mix salad. You know the mesclun greens? Well, I've hated it for years, ever since it became the most popular salad on the menu. And here's why. Unless you get your spring mix fresh from the farmer's market and use it that very same day, inevitably the red oak leaf lettuce wilts and rots and turns to black slime that clings to the other lettuces like gum on the bottom of your shoe. I can't bear it. Instead, give me romaine, arugula, baby spinach, watercress (my favorite), radicchio, endive, chicory, frisée, or Bibb. Or even nice red oak lettuce, fresh and eaten that same day, before it has a chance to melt down. But as for spring mix? It makes great compost.

Food values

There's a lot about pesticides and how they affect us that scientists don't yet know, but absence of knowledge is not proof of their safety. So use this list* of the fresh fruits and vegetables that consistently have the highest and lowest pesticide loads to help you decide how you're going to spend your produce dollars.

HIGHEST IN PESTICIDES	LOWEST IN PESTICIDES
Apples	Asparagus
Bell peppers	Avocados
Celery	Bananas
Cherries	Broccoli
Grapes	Cauliflower
Nectarines	Corn
Peaches	Kiwi fruit
Pears	Mangoes
Potatoes	Onions
Red raspberries	Papaya
Spinach	Pineapples
Strawberries	Peas

*Source: Environmental Working Group. Go to its website at www.foodnews.org to download a wallet-size produce shopping guide.

Making fresh produce last

There's one teensy-weensy problem with trying to eat more fruits and vegetables: They spoil. Quickly. We've all seen the sad end to our best intentions: soggy carrots, soft apples, spongy celery. Never fear. Where there's a will, there's a way, and Melissa is the queen of finding the way to make produce last and put veggies to work for you. Here are her tips:

- Wash and wrap the lettuce: As soon as possible—like right when you get home from the farmer's market or store—wash and dry all your salad greens. If you bought salad in a bag, rinse it anyway (see "Should You Bag the Bag?" page 86), but not until you want to use it. Then wrap the greens in a dish towel, put them in a plastic bag, and stick them in the vegetable crisper. They can keep up to a week stored this way.

- If you didn't take the advice above, refresh sad, wilted lettuce by soaking it in cold water for 20 minutes, then spin it dry and use it.

- Store sliced carrot sticks and celery sticks in water in the fridge.

- Don't ever wash berries until just before using; they rot really quickly once wet. If you need to wash them ahead of time for, say, a party, spread them out to dry on a dish towel-lined baking pan and then refrigerate.

- Store watercress and fresh herbs in a glass of water in the fridge.

- Many fruits and veggies (such as nectarines, peaches, and mangoes) can be refrigerated once they've ripened on the counter. Bananas too; although they turn black and look icky, they taste fine.

- When fruit is just beginning to go bad, cut it into chunks, remove the rotten/soft bits, and either freeze the rest to use in smoothies or cook it with a little sugar to make a compote to eat on yogurt for breakfast.

How (and how long) to store produce

FRUIT/VEGGIE	FRIDGE OR COUNTER?	HOW LONG WILL IT LAST?
Acorn Squash	Counter or a cool space like a pantry or cellar	Number of days or weeks
Apples (whole)	Counter or fridge	1 week on the counter, 2 weeks in the fridge
Arugula	Fridge	2 days
Avocado	Counter	2–5 days, depending on ripeness
Bananas	Counter, then fridge	3–5 days, plus an additional week
Blueberries	Fridge	7–10 days
Broccoli	Fridge	2–3 days
Cauliflower	Fridge	4–5 days
Celery	Fridge	7–10 days
Cucumber	Fridge	3–5 days
Grapefruit	Fridge	2 weeks
Mango	Counter, then fridge	2–3 days, plus an additional 3 days
Mesclun (spring mix)	Fridge	3 days
Nectarine	Counter, then fridge	2–3 days, plus an additional 5 days
Orange	Fridge	2 weeks
Peach	Counter, then fridge	2–3 days, plus an additional 5 days
Pepper	Fridge	7 days for red, 10 days for green
Red leaf lettuce	Fridge	3–5 days
Romaine lettuce	Fridge	5–7 days
Snap peas	Fridge	4–5 days
Spinach	Fridge	3–5 days
Sprouts	Fridge	3–4 days
Strawberries	Fridge	2–3 days
String beans	Fridge	4–5 days
Sweet potato	Counter or cool space like a pantry or cellar	1 week
Tomato	Counter	3 days to a week, depending on its ripeness and time of year
Watercress	Fridge	4–5 days
Zucchini	Fridge	3–4 days

Robin says:

When I started eating on The Skinny, *I started making a lot of broccoli for my kids at dinner (sauteed with a little garlic, salt, and olive oil). Both kids actually like broccoli, and it's way better for me to mooch their broccoli rather than their (organic) chicken nuggets.*

Melissa admits:

For me the constant battle with life on The Skinny *is keeping my sweet tooth at bay. Saying no to that second (OK, third) cookie is something I practice every single day. It does get easier though, as long as I remind myself that the cookie I didn't eat today will taste just as good tomorrow.*

So what else should you eat?

All right. You can't live on fruits and vegetables alone. You also need grains, fats, protein, shortbread (if you're Melissa), and chocolate chip cookies (if you're Robin). In other words, your daily diet should be fairly well-rounded. Eat what you want, but be conscious of the good and bad health consequences of foods. Here's how to think about accompanying your fruits and vegetables:

Protein

Your body needs protein for all kinds of functions. Fish, chicken, tofu, tempeh, seitan, beans, meat, eggs—these are protein-rich foods. Having protein—on top of a salad, in soup, alongside a big helping of lightly sauteed vegetables, along with your fruit—at most meals will help keep you satisfied longer. A good portion size is 6 ounces, or the size of the palm of your hand. Leaner proteins like chicken, fish, and tofu are a healthier choice than red meat and dairy. Limit your red meat to small (less than 6-ounce) portions no more than once or twice a week.

Whole grains

Eat them. We need grains. They have fiber, B vitamins, and more good stuff. Choose whole grains such as brown rice, multigrain bread, oats, barley, quinoa, and whole wheat couscous.

"White" (aka milled) grains

Be moderate. Limit white bread, white pasta, white rice, and other white flour products. You won't get the same nutritional benefits from "white" grains as from whole grains because white grains are milled in a process that strips away most of their fiber and vitamins. This leaves you with food that's quickly absorbed by the body, bringing on a sugar rush. When you eat processed grains, you get hungrier faster than you do with slow-moving, fiber-rich whole grains.

The very good fats

Eat them. These are plant-based fats that are known as monounsaturated fats. Healthwise, they increase your "good" cholesterol (HDL) and help lower the "bad" cholesterol (LDL). You can find them in nuts, olives, plant-based oils (canola, corn, olive, soybean, peanut, safflower, sesame), avocados, seeds (such as pumpkin, sesame, and sunflower), and tahini (made from ground sesame seeds).

The still-good fats

These nutritious and important polyunsaturated fats include omega-3 essential fatty acids. They are present in walnuts, walnut oil, salmon, flax, pumpkin seeds and their oil, soybeans and soybean oil, and purslane. They've been shown to be good for your heart as well as your skin and hair (and we know how you feel about your skin and hair).

ROBIN'S RHUBARB TRICK

So I'm talking to Melissa on the phone and it's late spring and I'm whining about rhubarb. I see piles of it at the farmer's market. I know I should make something with it because it's in season. But I also know if I buy it, it's going to sit in my fridge until it turns into brown, mucky water, and my husband will find it and say, "Can I just ask? Are you going to do something with this?" So Melissa says to me about the rhubarb (as I know she will), "Oh, that's easy!"

Here's her trick: Wash a pound of rhubarb, chop it up, and throw it in a pot with one-half cup sugar and a quarter cup of either orange juice or water. Cover and let it simmer until it's mushy. It won't take long—maybe 10 minutes. It's delicious!

Even with my two delightful critters (I mean children) clinging to my legs, I know I'll be able to do just what Melissa said, and then I'll be able to put it in a pie or mix it with some yogurt or serve it with some grilled meat. Taking the extra step to make this fruit work is just Not That Hard!

The bad fats (aka fatty fats)

Be moderate. These are saturated fats, the type that clogs your arteries. You'll find them in full-fat dairy products (such as butter, milk, whole-fat yogurt, and cottage cheese), mayonnaise, and creamy ranch dressings, which are often made with sour cream.

Butter is certainly not the best thing for you, and too much of it will eventually clog your arteries. But saturated fats are not as bad as trans fats (see below), which are what you'll find in margarine and vegetable shortenings like Crisco. So if you're faced with a bread spread, don't eat it. You're much better off with a little bit of the real deal.

Do we have to tell you to enjoy but go very easy on deep-fried foods? Fries, onion rings, fried chicken, fried calamari—how good is all that fatty food? So good you only need to have a little bit every so often.

Trans fats

Trans fats have been covered heavily by the news media for good reason: They're evil. Limit or banish trans fats, which increase your level of bad (LDL) cholesterol and decrease your level of good (HDL) cholesterol. They make blood platelets sticky, which increases the likelihood of blood clotting in your heart or brain. Those blood clots can lead to heart disease and strokes. If you're nursing? The trans fats go right through your milk and get a head start at clogging your baby's arteries. (Even if you're not nursing, that fact is appalling.)

Trans fats are in many processed foods, such as potato chips. So read the label. Trans fats should be listed, per government regulations. Watch for "partially hydrogenated vegetable oil" or "vegetable shortening," which are trans fats in linguistic disguise.

How much should you eat of each group?

We're not fans of telling you how many servings a day you should eat from any one food group. Eat reasonably, eat more fruits and vegetables, use your common sense, and acknowledge that humongous amounts of food mean humongous calories (and maybe not humongous nutrients). And if you want to know what the U.S. government says about serving sizes, go to www.mypramid.com.

You also know our spiel about portions: Control them (except for fresh fruits and nonstarchy vegetables, which you can eat in unlimited quantities).

To help you think about how to establish a routine of balanced eating, here are a couple of *Skinny* tricks:

Trick 1: Divvy up the plate in your head. Decide what you're going to eat half of, what you're going to eat two-thirds of, and what you're going to finish. (Like any dieting technique, it's a little crazy-making and a little liberating. See if you like it.)

Trick 2: Go halfsies. If you're not into divvying up, just have half of what's on the plate and take home the rest or leave it behind. (Melissa's mom does this and she's lost 85 pounds and counting.)

Trick 3: Walk the balance beam (see Chapter 11, page 129). This is true not only for "treats" but also for the basic food groups. In other words, if you had half a bagel for breakfast, don't have a slice of pizza for lunch. Instead, have a salad or big bowl of soup. If you had fruit and yogurt for breakfast, you don't need grilled cheese for lunch (that's too much dairy). Have hummus and veggies on a pita or wrap. You get the idea. Let your past meal help you gauge what to have at your next meal and, uh, don't forget to eat a lot of vegetables and fruit. (Check out our

DO YOU NEED DAIRY?

How much dairy we should eat—or whether we should eat it at all—is a subject of constant debate. On the negative side, dairy has heart-clogging fat, and it irritates some people's stomachs and immune systems. On the positive side, dairy has calcium and protein and is, generally speaking, yummy. So whether you should eat dairy or how much of it you should eat is really up to you.

Nondairy sources of calcium include broccoli, tofu, spinach, bok choy, mustard greens, dandelion greens, turnip greens, kale, rhubarb, almonds, legumes, and blackstrap molasses. You can also take a calcium supplement. Weight-bearing exercises such as running, yoga, and lifting weights done three times a week will also strengthen your bones.

"2-Week Meal Plan," page 227, to see how we suggest balancing out meals.)

Trick #4: Take a daily multivitamin. Whether or not the human body absorbs nutrients as well in pill form as it does from food may be debated forever. Still, a multivitamin is a good way to supplement your daily nutritional needs. Also consider taking a calcium supplement and an omega-3 essential fatty acid supplement (choose one that's guaranteed free of heavy metals and PCBs).

The Takeaway

- Eat vegetables. Eat fruit.
- Want a snack? Have a piece of fruit, some cherry tomatoes, or carrot sticks.
- Want some fries? Stanch your hunger first with salad. Eat more of the salad than the fries.
- Establish a balanced eating routine by including whole grains, lean proteins, and good fats in your daily meals.
- Yes, fruits and veggies are healthful, but they also taste really good. Enjoy what you eat!

Chapter 8

Ladies Who Lunch The Skinny Way

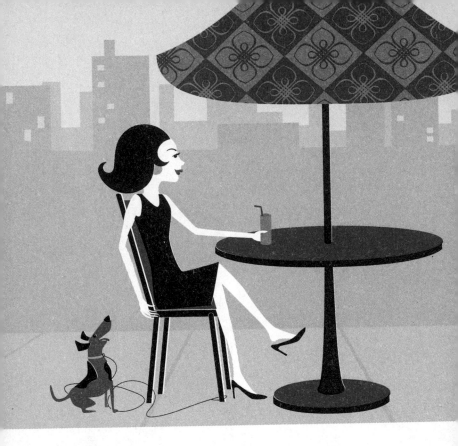

Let's lunch

When we dream about lunch, we imagine the kind we're sure Europeans have every day. You know, the lunch for which young boys in short pants sprint through cobblestone streets. The one where families relax for an hour (or more!) around a table eating only the freshest foods, perfectly prepared by a grinning, buxom grandma whose hands work magic on the humblest zucchini and eggplant. No, we don't often (or ever) get to enjoy those red-wine-in-a-water-glass lunches during the work week while we're toiling away, earning our daily bread and monthly shoes.

But it's not as though your choices are *either* the long, leisurely lunch *or* the soggy sandwich on the go. Lunch can be tasty, convenient, and *Skinny*, even on a workday. Ideally, it should be reasonably healthy and it should be filled with vegetables, fruit, and a mix of well-controlled portions of proteins, good fats, and whole grains.

Can't I eat what I want for lunch?

Of course you can eat what you want for lunch. But, like any time you eat, we strongly encourage you to figure out what you truly, most deeply, and madly want—and why. You must be even more aggressive and honest about your cravings during the working week than in your nonworking hours. Because when you're at work, it's all too easy to indulge for reasons that have less to do with what your body needs and more to do with the emotions and pressures of your day. Take these examples:

"My job is stressful; therefore, I must have a burrito with extra guacamole."
Even the best job brings its share of stress, but if you always eat to soothe the stress of work, well—we hate to break it to you—your little black dress is going to get a little bigger every year. When it comes to job stress, we must figure out a way to cope that doesn't involve anything deep-fried, frosted, or melted. Try breathing exercises, try finding a private room and do a headstand, try taking a walk around the block every two hours. Just don't try the newest candy bar at the newsstand.

"I'm having my weekly lunch with my work pals, and they're neither on The Skinny *nor skinny, but I still want what they're having. Besides, they'll notice if I'm eating something other than my usual cheeseburger deluxe."*
Do not eat a cheeseburger because of peer pressure. Yes, it's good. But you've had many of them, and you'll have more of them. Maybe you're going to have a scrumptious burger at dinner, or maybe once a month you'll tuck into the big beef at lunch. But once a week? With the fries? You don't need it, and you probably don't want it as much as you think you might. Too often, that big lunch feed (pizza, onion rings, whatever) has more to do with habit than desire.

"I'm bored at work."
That's OK, but it's not a good reason to have a whole Italian hero for lunch. Granted, you won't be bored while you're eating the hero, but you'll be so stuffed and dizzy and tired from all that meat and cheese and bread that you'll only get sleepier and more

bored as the afternoon drags on. Save yourself the trouble and have some melon instead.

All this to say: Unless it's a special occasion, and unless you are sure that what you have to have for lunch is that Fill-In-the-Blank-with-Something-Not-So-Healthy, don't waste your waist on a weekday lunch.

Office lunch: Bring it in, bring it on

There are all kinds of advantages to bringing in lunch.
Here are three:

1. **Ingredient control.** You always have more control over what goes into food you make. Wonder how much oil was slathered on those grilled vegetables in the gourmet food shop case? You don't need to guess when you grill them yourself. Do you want more Moroccan carrots and fewer red peppers? When you make it yourself, you decide how much of what goes where.

2. **Portion control.** When you pack what goes on the plate, you can easily keep it on the reasonable-size side.

3. **Money control.** Overall, you'll save money on food you make at home. Plus, you can allocate money toward special ingredients as you prefer. Free-range eggs, stinky cheese, wild salmon—you decide what ingredients are worth spending a few extra shekels for.

To be fair, there are three disadvantages to bringing your own lunch to work:

1. **Preparation.** You've got to do it in advance. Shop, cook, clean up, and pack up, when all you really want to do is hang out. It's time for an attitude adjustment: If you think of these things as chores, they're always going to be. If you think of them—especially the cooking part—as time spent taking care of yourself and learning about your foods, then maybe you'll get into cooking in a whole new way.

2. **You may not want it tomorrow.** So much of what we eat is determined by our whims, and our whims are all dictated by what's going on around us. (Did you smell that? Is someone having a slice of pepperoni pizza? Oh, I want pizza!) So how can you know if in 12 hours you'll still want that nice asparagus salad you made and packed tonight?

   All we can say is sometimes you can get what you want (store the salad in the fridge for the next day and buy a slice of pizza today). Other times you (forgive us) can get what you need (e.g., you're dining out that night, so eat the salad and skip the pizza).

3. **You give up an activity.** There's no denying that going out and buying lunch—picking out where you'll go, perusing the menu or salad bar, and getting the goods— adds a change of pace to your day. And when you bring your lunch, you say goodbye to that.

   Be positive! You can still eat with a friend, you can buy a nice cup of tea, and, with the time you save, you have many more minutes to blog-surf on your lunch hour. Never mind the shopping that can happen with the extra time and the moola saved by home cooking.

Brown bagging 101

Yes, packing your lunch is work. But we still think it's a good idea to bring lunch more often than not. Here are some *Skinny* tips to make it happen.

Grill in advance.

Robin has a friend who has a friend who'd buy salmon or chicken or tofu on Sundays, grill it up, and bring it with salad the rest of the week. This is a good strategy for lunches Monday through Thursday. Thursday night, though, it'll be time to defrost some soup for Friday's lunch—or you can plan on eating out that day.

What to grill: A protein. You can either grill a couple of small pieces of different things or a whole batch of one thing. Good choices include chicken (preferably skinless), salmon (the easiest fish to grill and store because it's thick and packed with good-for-you omega-3 essential fatty acids), or tofu. Flank steak is also a good pick, but you should limit red meat to once or twice a week. Your portion size for lunch should be about 4 ounces, which is the size of your closed fist. Don't worry about weighing things exactly; you can ask your butcher to cut up smallish pieces for you and work with what you have.

What to put it on: Watercress, arugula, spinach, mixed greens, or romaine.

Add in: Pumpkin seeds, sunflower seeds, walnuts, chickpeas, feta, roasted bell peppers, goat cheese, pear slices, whatever. Or nothing. A salad of protein over greens is simple and delicious.

What to put on it: Melissa makes the most delicious Caesar salad dressing (page 192). Try the Grainy Mustard Dressing (page 155), which is a happy complement to any protein. Or simply use good olive oil, a drizzle of lemon juice, and salt.

What else to grill: Vegetables. The best veggies to grill are zucchini, portobello mushrooms, onions, scallions, eggplant, bell peppers, and fennel. Before you grill, brush them with a little olive oil and season with salt and pepper. These can be served with a grilled protein or on greens with the add-ins (especially cheese, chickpeas, and/or nuts for some fat and protein) and maybe a little dressing. Or just pack them in a container and add a crusty piece of bread and a small(ish) piece of cheese.

Defrost

A nice hot bowl of soup with a fresh whole grain roll and/or small salad makes an excellent lunch. When you make soup, double the recipe and freeze half in individual-size (8-ounce) plastic containers so you can just grab and go. That way defrosting means simply taking out a container, wrapping it in a plastic bag, and putting it in your work tote before you leave for work. It will either fully or partially defrost by lunchtime and will, in any case, be fine after you heat it up.

The accoutrements

Just like accessorizing your little black dress, packing some extra tidbits to spice up your lunch can make the ordinary seem special. Bring in a small bag of sliced fennel, a couple of olives, or a handful of smoked almonds. Or go out and get yourself a fresh whole grain roll. These things will make you happy. If you must, must, must have chips, eat half of the bag and throw the rest in a garbage can far away from your workspace. You could also toss half the chips before you start to eat.

Heading out

So you're not packing it in today; you're heading out for lunch. If you're turning to your stolid survivors—sandwich, soup, or salad—consider these points:

The sandwich

Sandwiches are wonderful things. But, like a bowl of cereal in the morning, it's easy to fall into a sandwich rut. Turkey on rye, tuna on whole wheat, egg salad on sourdough. They're go-tos, standbys, easy-peasy, and they can be extremely satisfying—if you like sandwiches, that is.

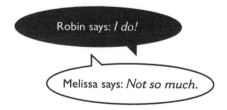

Robin says: *I do!*

Melissa says: *Not so much.*

We say: If you want a sandwich, have a sandwich (or have half now, half later). But be mindful of their pitfalls:

1. They get soggy.

2. They often contain mayonnaise, which is unfriendly to a weight loss endeavor and a little hard to track. A tuna

salad sandwich may not feel like a huge lunch, but it does pack a bad-fat punch. (As an alternative, check out the mayo-free tuna recipe, Tuna and Cucumber Salad with Olives, page 170.)

3. Fabulous sandwiches from nifty little shops tend to be overstuffed. Often they're stuffed with great things that can be hard to keep in stock at home—sun-dried tomatoes, tapenade, Gouda—and sometimes you want those things. But how often have you stared at the gaping maw of a ciabatta roll stuffed with yellow curried chicken salad and arugula? Or the you-swear-it-could-be-a-whole-breast-of-turkey with provolone, roasted pepper, and arugula on a baguette? *The Skinny* idea is this: If the sandwich can't be easily closed or easily held in one hand, take out about half the stuffing. It's too much. You don't need it. Really.

The soup

Soup is excellent food. It's high volume for its calories, which means you can eat a lot of it, feel quite full, get a lot of nutritional bang, and not blow a whole day's worth of treats in one sitting. Choose brothy soups, vegetable soups, hearty bean soups, and even big-noodle soups over any "cream of" soup or cream-based chowder.

The salad

Anything that's on a plate, has something to do with vegetables, or isn't stuck between two pieces of bread can be defined as a salad. A perfect salad mixes the unexpected with the understood (Citrus Salad with Fennel, Olives, and Onions, page 159), the exuberant with the restrained (Celery Salad with Blue Cheese and Tabasco, page 162). If you're having the salad for an entire meal, it must include a protein, a fat, and a big mound of vegetables, all of which will help you get full and stay full. But not all salads are a dieter's delight. There are issues.

1. **All dressed up.** If someone tosses your salad for you, odds are the tosser is going to put way too much dressing on it. This isn't just a calorie issue (although

dressing is full of high-calorie stuff like olive oil, mayo, and sour cream). It's also a taste issue: Your fresh vegetables are getting smothered! Let them breathe! Ask your salad maker to use half the amount he or she usually does. Or ask for your own little container of dressing and be sure not to use more than half of it.

2. A "salad" isn't always a salad. You know this. Throw in cheese and ham and bacon and pasta and more cheese and just because it's called a salad doesn't mean it'll rest lightly on your abdomen. If you have a salad that's just bursting with stuff (and not that many vegetables), remove some of it.

3. A salad can be filling. (So stop eating.) Sometimes when you have a salad—a nice, mannered, protein-and-fat-portion-controlled salad—you feel so proud, so righteous, that it's hard to believe you're full. It's hard to accept that you don't have to eat more now or shouldn't have a big honking blondie for dessert. After all, all you had was a salad. And it didn't have bacon.

But unless you're dying for the blondie, you know why not. (Don't have it just to have it or because it's there or because you always have it.) It can be hard to get used to the idea that a salad is enough food, but it is.

Melissa says:

Good salad bars—the kind with plenty of crisp vegetables, tasty dressings, some nice croutons, and quality cheeses—are my favorite way to eat lunch. A salad bar lets me tailor my own salad—but all the shopping, washing, peeling, and slicing has been done for me, and the variety of vegetables simply makes me giddy. I can cherry pick and get exactly what I'm in the mood for, even if it's a little offbeat: baby arugula, string beans, hard-boiled eggs, sunflower seeds, marinated artichoke hearts. Or spinach, bacon, feta cheese, and beets with a little steamed broccoli. It's all good, easy, quick, and supersatisfying. (Note: If you chance upon the scary kind of salad bar that's mostly fried foods sitting under heat lamps, with a few wilted vegetables and suspect containers of canned corn and sliced olives bobbing in murky liquid, flee!)

The power lunch

The power lunch is a form of business lunch. It often takes place at a nice restaurant. During such a lunch, your food choices are dictated not only by what you want but also by the weird assumptions and judgments that are part of the nonverbal communications of business dealings.

You might think that because you're at a power lunch, you have to order Man Food such as steak. You don't. The only thing that matters at a power lunch is how you order. Order with conviction. Unless the meeting is quite collegial, do not ask your server to tell you which is better, the sauteed trout or the Cobb salad. Choose for yourself.

No matter what you decide to eat, the ability to make a decision unapologetically and without flourish is the most important part of your meal. If you only want a salad of mixed greens, do not say, "I'll just have the mixed greens." Say, "I'll have the mixed greens, thanks." That "just" signals abstemiousness. If you're going to have the four-cheese ravioli, ask for it simply and do not shrug your shoulders with glee or resignation.

You may think all this direction about body language at lunch is beside the point of *The Skinny*, but we're all about feeling confident and good in your body, and at a power lunch that's precisely how you want to feel.

Whether you finish what you order is neither here nor there, but you must eat some of it. If you stop eating before you've finished the entire dish, do so without comment. Be powerful and serene.

Brunch: The most dangerous meal

Brunch is a meal that makes people insane. There's something both decadent and comforting about it. You know exactly what's going to be on the menu: French toast (challah!), eggs any way (and bacon!), buttermilk pancakes (you can't make them like that without a griddle!).

Cro-Magnon man and woman must have gone to brunch. Why else do we all respond so positively to this meal? Why else would otherwise reasonable people wait 45 minutes for a cup of coffee if the experience wasn't hardwired somewhere in our prehistoric shared memory?

Of course, there's the food. It covers our basic desires for sweet and salty and greasy. If you're at a brunch place or a home brunch worth its salt, the servings will be enormous. If you're combining breakfast and lunch, after all, you get to double up on the servings too, right?

Maybe. Let's say it's a Sunday morning, after you've slept off your night in your little black dress, and you're ready to sit down and dig into a big meal. Is it worth it to you to consider the implications of this meal on your waistline?

You may be a little tired, a little hungover, or a little excited about getting a table at the great brunch joint. You don't want to be thinking about portion size or healthy choices or whether you should have the whole bagel or half. You want what you want.

You want our *Skinny* advice? OK, here it is:

1. Skip the muffins entirely, no matter how mini, unless that's what you really want for brunch.

2. If something comes with fresh fruit or greens on the side, get them. And eat them.

3. Good home fries are rare. Nine times out of 10 they're mediocre. Skip 'em and stick with the whole grain toast.

ROBIN'S FAVORITE BRUNCH

The brunch I look forward to most each year is Melissa's birthday brunch. She buys a slew of smoked fish from Russ & Daughters in Manhattan and serves it alongside salads that are So Good they actually hold my interest.

It's always a very festive affair, this brunch, and all of her friends, many of whom haven't seen each other since last year's brunch, have a swell time catching up over the salads and salmon, which let you have half a bagel and not feel deprived. (Though since it's once a year, I often have a whole bagel, dammit.) She also gets doughnuts from this fancy pants place, Doughnut Plant, where the doughnuts are sublime.

Except for the coffee (Melissa is a tea drinker and her coffee is disgusting), it is the perfect brunch.

4. Do not finish the pancakes or French toast. Stop eating when there's a reasonable amount left. (If you ordered three pancakes, leave one or more depending on their size; ditto for the French toast.) If you can't stop picking, pawn your leftovers off on someone else at the table.

5. Have half a bagel. (One bagel is the equivalent of five servings of whole grains. Distressing, isn't it?) While you may know people who scoop out a bagel's doughy filling, we urge you to leave your half intact. Give yourself a reasonable shmear of cream cheese (not too big, not too small; if you're measuring, a scant tablespoon) and then pile it as high with smoked salmon and whitefish as you like. Why be so generous with the fish portions? So often we (as in Robin and Melissa) want to have a second half of bagel not for the bread but as a conveyor for more smoked fish. By piling the fish on one bagel half, we get more fish (good) and less bread.

6. If you're at a buffet, serve yourself once and do not go back for seconds. And no mini muffins!

If you decide you're going to finish the pancakes or have a whole bagel or—damn us—have those muffins, you know the rest of the day's meals should be somewhat compensatory and restrained. A big salad, a brothy soup, a grilled chicken breast. And for goodness' sake, once you've digested, get some exercise! Take a walk, a bike ride, a run, a yoga class—something. Just move your booty.

The Takeaway

- Make lunch simple.
- Make lunch flavorful.
- Don't make too much of lunch.
- Skip the fries and forget about the club sandwich. Make lunch work for you.
- If it's brunch, choose your poison.

Chapter 9

Let's Do Dinner

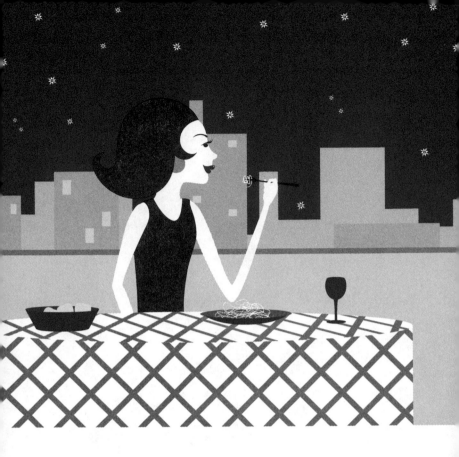

Out on the town

There you are, all decked out in your little black dress and Sigerson Morrison boots, with dinner reservations at the hottest place in town and your sweetie on your arm. You feel great, you look great, you know the restaurant will be great. Maybe someone else is footing the bill, or it's your night for a well-deserved splurge.

Isn't this the time to toss *The Skinny* caution to the wind? Do you really need to order a salad?

Well, no and yes. And vice versa.

By now you know that being on *The Skinny* is all about eating what you want when you really, really want it. So the question you need to ask yourself before you order the foie gras-stuffed beef tenderloin with half-butter-half-potato puree is, "Is this really what I want, right now?"

Eating dinner out is almost always about three things: novelty, companionship, and excess. Often a meal out means you'll be offered a lot of food, much of which you haven't had exactly that way before. (Even a grilled steak is different depending on where you get it.) You'll be sharing the experience with at least one other person. It will be, if not a full-on little-black-dress-worthy occasion, at least somewhat special because, well, you're eating out. And unless you're Melissa and you eat out for a living, you don't get to eat out every night.

So there you are, confronted by a tempting array of dishes. What will you do with it all? Your choices will have a lot to do with (a) how good the food is, (b) your mood, expectations, and cravings, and (c) your relationship with your dinner date(s).

The big picture

By now you know *The Skinny*'s overall approach to meal eating:

1. Eat what you want, and don't eat what you don't want. For restaurants, this translates into: Order what you want, but don't eat what you don't want just because it came on the plate next to what you do want.

2. Pay attention to your food. Slow down, appreciate, and savor.

3. Enjoy your food. Make sure that every bite is contributing to your overall happiness. Otherwise, proceed to #4.

4. Stop eating when you've had enough. That's more for Robin, less for Melissa. Learn to tell how much is enough for you.

So there you are. No problem! The next time you find yourself out at a restaurant that's doing its job well by enticing you with food you wouldn't, or couldn't, make at home, in serving sizes you'd likely divide into three (two meals, one snack), you'll fully enjoy everything you eat—and you'll leave at least a little bit behind on the plate.

You won't let your fork wander to your mouth unheeded. You won't eat too quickly or forget to slow down so you can figure out if you're done.

You won't worry about wasting money or food. And you won't be concerned about what your dinner companion(s) will think or say (either to your face or behind your back) about what you are or are not eating.

You won't agree to share a dessert you don't really want and then eat most of it.

You won't drown your taste buds in a third Cosmopolitan because you know you'll be tempted to say, "Enough of *The Skinny*. Right now, I'm on the Cosmy."

Right?

Actually, eventually, yes.

Practice makes skinny

You might not believe it, but as you practice a little restraint each time you eat out, sooner than you think, you'll probably find yourself satisfied with smaller portions. And pretty soon after that, you'll find that even when you're eating out, eating smaller and pickier feels happier and natural.

Because how you eat is all about how you're used to eating.

ROBIN'S NEW PIZZA PHILOSOPHY

The longer I've been living *The Skinny*, the more I notice I don't always want what I assumed I'd always want.

Take pizza. Just the other day, we were at a gathering of neighbors where pizza was served. I chose my slice (ricotta and spinach) and thought maybe I'd have a slice of the meat-lover's pizza next. I ate the first slice, then ate some salad, and then realized I didn't really want a second piece.

This made me a little dizzy.

I saw that my husband was having a slice of the meat-lover's pizza, so I asked him for a bite. It was fine, but I didn't want more. I had some more salad, and I was happy. A little shocked, but satisfied.

I'll be honest, I really thought Melissa was just being a nutty size-2 Melissa with that "one slice" thing, but she wasn't. There will be a time when I want a second slice (such as when I'm face-to-face with my absolute all-time favorite eggplant-and-pepperoni pie). But for just your average pizza? Melissa is right: One piece may just be enough.

We're not saying to always eat less; we're just saying to give yourself a minute before you eat more.

This book won't be of use to you if you say, "Tomorrow I'll eat half my bagel and throw the other half away, have a big salad for lunch, skip the cookies, only have three fries at the restaurant for dinner because I'll really want those fries, and then eat only half of the dessert I want most of all."

While this is a version of what we advocate (except for the no cookies and the counting of fries), it's too extreme for day one. It's like you decided to take swimming lessons and jumped into the deep end of the pool. You can try it, but you might just get too frustrated and reject the whole thing (or at least get water up your nose).

Instead scale back a little here and a little there until scaled-back eating seems perfectly natural.

This is especially important when you eat out because of these special challenges restaurant meals create:

1. You're paying good money for your meal and you want your money's worth.

2. What you're having is so good, and you'd never make it at home.

3. You don't want to talk diet talk with your dinner companion and you certainly don't want to have to come up with a snappy, on-the-spot response to his/her Big Idea of, "C'mon, let's just share the fried chicken, mac 'n' cheese, and jalapeño poppers!"

4. If you usually do talk diet talk with this particular dinner companion, then you don't want to get into a whole, competitive "Who can eat less?" thing. Who needs that?

5. How often do you get to eat out?

6. One/some/all of the above.

All this to say, give yourself time to get used to eating a different way.

Practice Steps

Yes, dinner out on *The Skinny* takes practice. Use these tips to cut back on one aspect of your meal at a time.

First time out: Avoid what you like least

You may already do this without even noticing. For example, when Robin eats breakfast out, she often orders two eggs over easy with toast. That dish almost always comes with home fries, and she can't remember the last time she had more than a forkful of home fries. Which is to say, decide what on your plate is your home fry and only warrants a bite or two and leave the rest.

When Melissa's out at a fancy work dinner and has to order three full courses, she always orders one dish that doesn't really appeal to her at that moment. So taking a few tastes and leaving the rest isn't hard because she's either not in the mood for the liver-and-onion entrée or she ordered something she doesn't particularly love, like the seared chicken breast (which always seems dry to her). This makes it easy to finish whatever she wants to finish and to leave the thing she likes the least. Try this once, then repeat.

Another time out: Have more of what you like most

Figure out what you want the most in each course. We don't just mean what you've ordered; if there's more than one basic element to the dish you're being served, and if it doesn't have to all be eaten together, decide where you're not going to hold back.

For us this is especially useful when it comes to dessert. If you get a dessert that has ice cream and bread pudding, have a little of both, and then make the decision: Tonight, is it the ice cream or the bread pudding? Another night it may be the bread pudding, but tonight it's the ice cream.

Focus your attention on the ice cream and leave some of the bread pudding behind—even if it's one last bite. We know leaving one lonely bite on the plate can seem absurd. Why not just have it? But it's not absurd because it's not about that last little bit; it's about practicing having your (very satisfying) fill without having it all.

Next time out: Veggies first

So you know how to evaluate your menu choices and negotiate between what you want the most and least. You can leave behind even a little of something you like in order to have more of something you love. These are important strategies for *Skinny* maintenance and should be followed as often as possible.

If you eat out a lot (like Melissa) or if you want to lose weight, it's time to start eating more veggies when you're out too. Order an appetizer that's veggie-heavy (and lightly dressed) or make sure to get a veggie side dish. Something nonstarchy and green is usually good: Try broccoli, string beans, snow pea pods, spinach.

If you know you're going to have the frozen chocolate hazelnut dessert, fill up on a lot of veggies during your appetizer and main course. Then acknowledge how full you are from your high-volume veggies before you finish the whole dessert.

THE PITFALLS OF FAMILY STYLE

"Family-style" restaurant meals can be dangerous. The food is just sitting there, and it's really, really hard to stop eating because it won't go away unless you make it go away (i.e., down your gullet). You start poking the corner of the chicken, or you slice away one extra sliver from the pizza, or you take one more half a serving spoon of stew. It's endless. Here's what to do:

- Take what you want from the serving dishes and then move the platters to the other side of the table, beyond the reach of your fork.

- If it's not polite to move the food away and you feel the need to pick at something, pick at the salad or vegetables.

- If the vegetables or salads are smothered in cheese, or if they're deep fried and there's no possibility of ordering anything like a plain green salad (say you're at a BBQ joint and the lightest thing on the menu is an order of fried green tomatoes), find the thing on the table that you want the most and put a small serving of that on your plate. Very slowly, pick at what's in front of you.

- If all else fails, busy your hands until the table is cleared. The picking has as much to do with wanting to keep your hands busy as anything else. Tap out "Chopsticks" on your leg, tell a joke that requires much gesticulating, or, you know, sit on them.

(Note: If the restaurant has a separate dessert menu, ask to see it with the main menu so you can figure out how to pace your meal; if there's nothing you want for dessert, you'll know you can eat more of your entrée.)

Forever after: Take your tasting menu seriously

When you order the prix fixe, multicourse tasting menu, taste, do not chow down. Don't finish everything on your plate. It's simply too much food. This is advice not just for *Skinny* living but for living, period. And it's not just about weight.

Many years ago, Melissa and Robin went to a dim sum brunch at a fancy New York restaurant. It had something like 12 courses.

MELISSA MAKES IT SMALL

When dining out I cut up my food into small pieces. I do this when I'm full after the appetizer but I don't really want to let on that I'm not eating all that much of dinner. Cutting the food up and moving it around the plate makes not eating much less obvious. It's a trick, and it works for me.

Robin has never done this. She's never been full after an appetizer and always wants to eat some of her dinner. But if you're full after your appetizer, and there's more food on the way, saw away! You never know what'll work for you.

Robin finished most of each course, Melissa, not so much. Afterwards, Melissa went shopping with her boyfriend, and Robin stumbled home in a daze and lay on her bed until the next day. No Sunday laundry, no finishing the novel she'd been hankering to get to. None of it. Nada. Zilch. Just digesting. That's no fun.

The dinner companion

In Chapter 8, "Ladies Who Lunch *The Skinny* Way," we talked about the challenges that can arise when lunching with colleagues. Whom we eat with has a huge influence on what we eat. There's how we feel about the person, there's how the person makes us feel, there's the shared history with food, there's the shared history with weight and body image and how that's played out in this particular relationship. All of this affects what we eat, how much we eat, and how we feel about both the food and the volume.

When you sit down to eat with someone who is not food neutral, identify what you want and support yourself first; try to establish workable boundaries between you and your friends and family members. Choose your location and your meal carefully if you want to lose weight and that's going to be an issue with your dining companion.

If you're meeting someone who might arch her eyebrows at a soup and salad for dinner, meet for coffee instead—or lunch. No one can scoff at soup and salad for lunch. Lunch is much less loaded (so to speak) than dinner when it comes to eating for fun because after it you have to continue with your day. You can always say you have a lot to do and if you load up on onion rings you'll only get sleepy.

If dinner is inevitable, choose a restaurant that doesn't advertise its enormous portions on the menu. ("Try our famous 16-ounce burger!") And if the subject of what you're eating comes up, and if it's not about how good the food is, change the subject. Don't get sucked into a black hole of food/body talk if you don't want to.

There are all sorts of things about how a dinner companion acts that you can't control, but you can have a say in where you eat, what you eat, and what you talk about.

LOVE IN MEAL TIME

We haven't really talked about how you negotiate changing your eating habits when you live with someone. We know it's complicated. We know it helps to have that person on board. We know it's hard when food—and we're not talkin' vegetables—is foreplay. We know that change, particularly change having to do with how you look and feel and what you weigh, can be scary to both you and your partner for many reasons.

A lover might like your curves (more than you do) or might be in no mood to consider changing his or her eating habits or to question how healthy his or her lifestyle is. A partner might want things to stay put when you're ready to shake them up.

It's serious business. Let's hope your sweetie is on board with your choices and supports you in them. But whatever your partner's position on your weight, you have to feel good about your choices, about why you're making them, and about what you want for yourself now and in the future.

Three dinners and a plan

Sometimes we find ourselves in dining situations that require a bit of delicate negotiating. Here are three, along with tips.

Dinner 1: You're out and you're starving! What to do?

- Take a deep breath.

- Have a piece of bread with a lot of butter (bread with butter sates your hunger better than bread alone).

- Drink a glass of water.

- Pace yourself, pace yourself, pace yourself.

- Don't order a huge meal just because you're so hungry now.

- Remember: Food is on the way.

Dinner 2: You're out but you're not hungry. What to do?

This happens to Melissa much more often than it does to Robin. Because (a) Melissa doesn't seem to get as hungry as Robin and (b) Melissa goes out all the time. (Nice work if you can get it.)

- Order as light a meal as you can. If you can get away with salad only, do so.

- If you must order two courses, order something you want for an appetizer and something that isn't that appealing as a main course. That way, you can eat some of what you'd like under any circumstance but not too much of anything when you're really not hungry anyway.

- Order something that you might like for lunch tomorrow. In other words, plan on asking for a doggie bag.

- Take this hint from Melissa: Ask your date for a bite or two of the fatty, rich, yummy thing he ordered that you sort of wish you'd ordered. A bite or two of mac and cheese can go a long way in between nibbles of your watercress-fennel salad.

Dinner 3: You're out but you want to be in. What to do?

This is a dangerous situation because when you find yourself in a restaurant when you really want to be home in bed, you'll be sorely tempted to order the most creamy, cheesy, fried, big-comfort-food thing on the menu. After all, if you can't be comforted by your comforter, food is the next best thing. Isn't it?

- Not really. If you don't want to be out, don't compound the situation by eating a lot of something that's not all that healthy and that may make you feel crappy later. Save your big meal splurge for when you're really happy and excited to be out. Eat a healthy, simple meal instead.

Embrace the doggie bag

Melissa takes food home from practically every restaurant she goes to. Not only does it caress the chef's ego (if the chef is even paying attention) because it means you liked the food enough to want to take it home, but leftovers make tasty lunches the next day—bulked out with salad, of course.

The other kind of dinner out: holiday meals

When you confront a holiday table groaning under the weight of dish after dish, be very thoughtful. Assess the full range of your choices. Think about the cook, decide what's likely to be best and what you want the most, and plan accordingly.

A TIP ON THE BILL

So you've ordered a salad and a glass of wine, and your charming companion has a steak and two martinis. How do you pay that bill if you don't want to split it down the middle? A gracious companion will offer to cover her part of the meal. If no such offer seems to be forthcoming, take a deep breath and say, "Oh, can I see the bill? Hmmm, it looks like I owe $XX. Plus tip, that's $XX." Be as straightforward as you can and don't make a big to-do about not paying for what you didn't eat.

While some people would say eat more of the simply and lightly prepared foods, we suggest you figure out the three things you want the most, and the one thing you want most of all, and give yourself portions accordingly.

Remember to take a lot of salad or the least fatty veggie you can find. Do this especially if you're really hungry or feel like you need to eat a lot because it's a special occasion (even though there's no rule that says you must eat a lot on a holiday) or because your cousin is crowing about her new Mini Cooper and Manolo Blahniks and you would like to drown her voice out with your own chewing.

Remember, when you eat what you want, you really don't need to eat a big pile of it to be satisfied by it.

Remember, dessert will be out soon, so pace yourself.

Remember not to hover by the buffet or, if you're seated at a table, not to pick (too much) at the platters of food before you (see page 113).

Finally, remember that every meal is about checks and balances. If you're going to go for the pecan pie, think twice about the full serving of mashed potatoes.

MELISSA ON THE DINNER PARTY

Throwing a dinner party at home has a lot in common with dining out—notably, my tendency to pig out. When I'm cooking, I'm nibbling, tasting, and munching constantly. By the time I sit down at the table with my guests, I am not at all hungry. I've probably already consumed twice as much as my normal meal's worth, and I'm totally sick of the flavors I've been nibbling, bite by bite, off the wooden spoon in the kitchen. This doesn't make me particularly happy. I want to enjoy the yummy dinner I cooked for my friends.

My solution? I try to make as much of the meal a day or two before. That way all my tasting has been done far ahead and by the time I sit down to dinner, I'm hungry for those flavors again. In winter, I favor stews and braised dishes that are even better when made a day or two ahead. Cold roasted meats are terrific in the summertime when served the next day.

The Takeaway

- Eating dinner out can be like eating any other meal on *The Skinny*. Practice eating what you like and not eating what you don't like.

- Don't worry about what your companions (or your server, the chef, or your date) will think about what you have or haven't eaten. Focus on yourself, your needs, and your desires.

- If you can, order something with fruits and/or vegetables.

- Stop eating when you're satisfied. And be honest with yourself about when that is.

- Bring leftover food home.

- Enjoy your food.

Chapter 10

The Skinny on Drinks

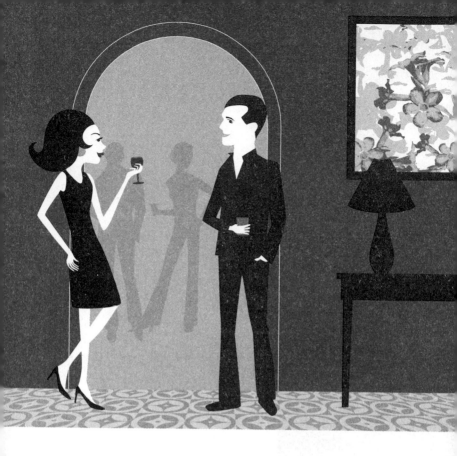

Skinny girls drink up

How wonderful it is to slake one's thirst. The cool relief of lemonade on a sultry afternoon; the aromatic bitterness of good, strong coffee in the morning; the icy, bracing first sip of a martini. The delights of drink are many and multifaceted.

Most of us don't think of drinks as affecting our pant size. Aside from a pounding headache the morning after one too many martinis, any downside to a drink (no matter the alcohol content) seems utterly beside the point. It all goes down so smoothly, so easily, so happily.

But juice, milk, smoothies, Cosmopolitans, wine, and, especially, frappuccinos all have calories. You may be surprised to learn that, on average, Americans get 21 percent of their calories from drinks.

If you're watching what you eat to lose or maintain weight, you can undermine a perfectly reasonable day of eating with a bottle of sweet iced tea here and some beer there. So if you're ready to get on *The Skinny*, it's time to pay attention to what you drink.

Daytime drinking

From now on, consider any drinks with calories to be in the same category as food. Don't sneak them in, pretending they don't count. And consider these *Skinny* tips.

For the righteous
If you're trying to lose weight, stick to water (flat or sparkling, with a squeeze of lemon or orange or whatever), and tea and coffee (iced or hot, but sweeten it yourself and add your own milk). If you like tea and coffee with a lot of milk, use fat-free. If only whole milk will do, limit yourself to three cups a day.

For the frothy hot drink lover
If your preferred hot drink is a latte, cappuccino, or a luscious, caramel macchiato, switch to regular coffee with milk while you're trying to lose weight. (We shouldn't have to tell you to skip the whipped cream.) When you hit your goal weight and you're in maintenance mode, the latte/cappuccino may return to your menu, but start ordering a smaller size—and, of course, try it at least once with fat-free milk.

Chai lattes taste like pure sugar—whether made with soymilk or cow's milk—and should be placed in the same category as a cookie. Which do you want more? The latte or the cookie?

On *The Skinny*, it's OK to have what you want, as long as you're honest with yourself about what it is you're eating. For example, a chai latte is not neutral when it comes to weight management. If you want to lose weight, and the lattes are not essential to your overall happiness, skip 'em.

Here's the exception: If you absolutely love your latte, or if the idea of saying no to cappuccino means doing something that feels only like deprivation, then don't do it. But get those lattes skinny (that is, with fat-free milk) and cut back somewhere else if you're trying to drop a few pounds—because the Balance Beam (Chapter 11) applies to drinks as well.

FRAME OF REFERENCE

We know, we know, we know: We don't count calories. But to give you a little frame of reference, here are some calorie counts from Starbucks latte-land:

Tall (12-ounce) whole-milk latte: 200 calories

Grande (16-ounce) whole-milk latte: 260 calories

Venti (20-ounce) whole-milk latte: 340 calories

Compare these with a 1.9-ounce Milky Way (the average size bar), which contains 228 calories; a 2.07-ounce package of Starburst, with 234 calories; and a 2-ounce Snickers with 273 calories.

Source: The Calorie Counter at www.thecaloriecounter.com

For those who hear the siren song of pretty bottles

In their smartly styled bottles filled with brightly colored liquids, these sirens sing out so prettily from the refrigerated case. There's the lip-puckering lemonade and the upscale juicy soda. There are Italian sodas that are both sweet and nicely acid-sharp, perfect on a hot day. And all those bottled sweetened teas.

If you want to lose weight, these are good choices if and only if one of them is the thing you want the most. Do you have to have the sparkling Italian soda? Have it with a salad. Does the cranberry juice beckon you at snack time? Say so long to the chips and have some carrots or an orange instead. Fruit juice has some of the nutritional benefits of regular fruit, but not all. Most notably, it's missing the fiber that slows digestion and helps you feel fuller longer. When you drink fiber-free fruit juice you're basically drinking sugar, even when you're getting freshly squeezed juice. If you really want the juice, have the juice, but keep in mind it's sweet because there's sugar in it.

If you decide you're going to have the flavored juicy juice drink, have it, but remember to check your portions: Odds are the bottle in your hands holds two servings, so double the calories listed on the label. Pour a cup of the stuff for now and put the rest away for another day.

For fruit smoothie fanatics

Filling, nutritious, and very satisfying to the sweet-toothed, fruit smoothies are great when you make them yourself. (Try the Almond Butter and Strawberry Breakfast Smoothie, page 152.) But when you buy one at the smoothie shack, check the ingredients list closely. At Robin's old gym, they made smoothies with frozen yogurt. After a good workout, you could end up drinking what's basically a fruity milk shake. So proceed with smoothie, but proceed with caution.

For athletes

If you do sports, you could gulp down sports drinks to replenish your electrolytes. By sports, we don't mean competitive shopping. We mean regular activities in which you exert yourself for more than 30 minutes. We mean you sweat profusely.

If you don't work out a couple of hours a day or train for a triathlon or road race on a regular basis, you're probably not losing electrolytes, which are restored by those sports drinks. Those drinks also serve up a boatload of sugar. (There are two servings in one bottle of Gatorade; check the label on other sports drinks.)

If you're thirsty after a workout or a long day, have some water and fruit. And if you're hungry, get yourself a well-balanced meal. But if you're thirsty after a 30-mile bike ride or running a marathon, have whatever you want!

ROBIN'S SKINNY MORNING JUICE

When I went to college, I stopped having orange juice in the mornings. (In fact, after an unfortunate night with vodka and orange juice, I stopped drinking orange juice altogether for about 10 years.) But when my husband and I first lived together, he made my breakfast every morning—as in, he poured out my cereal and a glass of juice, usually grapefruit. It was a sweet gesture, and it got me back into the juice habit.

When I went on *The Skinny*, I decided I'd mix the now-compulsory morning grapefruit juice with water. Not that full-on grapefruit juice is so bad, but I thought, why not? I actually think it makes the drink lighter and more refreshing. Orange juice, which is sweeter and thicker (and has more calories), needs to be cut with sparkling water, and that, to me, feels a bit much for first thing in the morning. Kind of like wearing your little black dress to meet someone for coffee. But grapefruit juice cut with water? If you're a morning juice junkie, try it.

A WORD ABOUT DIET SODA

We're not huge fans of diet soda. It leaves us feeling like we want more of something, and we're not sure what, so we end up grazing randomly and feeling kind of funky. We also feel a little funny about all the ingredients in them that we can't pronounce. But we also know that many people have strong feelings for and about their diet sodas, and so we're not going to make any big deal about them. If you really like them, have them. If you think they're just OK but find yourself ordering them because you think they're good for your diet, try skipping them and have home-brewed unsweetened iced tea or sparkling water with lemon instead.

Drinks by night

Here are some facts about alcoholic drinks—good, bad, and indifferent. There's sugar in alcohol, which means there are calories, so drink what you like, but keep in mind those calories add up quickly. Whatever the social situation, here are some moves for navigating the alcohol jungle so you can have your drink and dinner too.

The dive bar

There you are, out in your perfect Earl denim capris and brand-spanking-new little black top. You're meeting friends for drinks at the corner dive bar.

Here's what we'd drink: Bourbon. Straight up or spiked with some seltzer, water, or ice. A reasonably good bourbon is usually on the shelf of any bar, and it comes without the intensity of, say, a 12-year-old Scotch. It's satisfying in the mouth and a little goes a long way. More to the point, a glass of bourbon will have fewer calories than a cocktail made with fruit juices or liqueurs. Plus, we like it.

Here's what we don't drink: Beer. Drinking beer is like eating a meal. A good beer is chewy and satisfying. But there's a reason it feels hefty. It is. Hops, malt, amber waves of grain—it's all in there. If you want beer, have it, but skip the bread at dinner.

The fancy lounge

You've just perched your little-black-dressed frame on a supermod chair at the hippest lounge bar in town and, if you love an icy cocktail, this is your moment. Seize it. But bear in mind that generally, the simpler and more sophisticated the cocktail, the fewer the calories. Froufrou concoctions with apple vodka, juice, sorbet, or chocolate-hazelnut liqueur and cream may taste terrific and look swell, but they are more of a dessert than a beverage. If you like martinis, Cosmos, and Manhattans, stick to those.

GIVING UP THE GHOST

Two things happen when you drink: Your taste buds dull and your self-control loosens. The latter has all sorts of implications that we don't have to engage right now. The one we will engage is the Nacho Moment.

You've downed one margarita or two beers and there they are, the nachos, right in front of you. If you weren't feeling a little woo-woo-woo, you might not have even ordered them in the first place. But you were, and there they are.

In this situation, it's very hard to sit on your hands. It's very hard not to eat. You must make a choice.

If trying to stop when you know you've had enough will require a great deal of effort that will breed guilt and resentment, then don't do it. Give in to your nacho dreams and accept that tomorrow there will be fruit and whole grain toast and salad. Because once you move from "I'm eating and drinking and having fun" to "I'm eating and drinking and having fun and feeling like crap because of how much I've eaten," then, really, it's no fun. *The Skinny* rule? Avoid feeling like crap and maximize the fun.

We're not saying go wild all the time. We're saying if, every so often, you find yourself out with your old friend Margarita and her boyfriend Nacho Supreme, and if the fight against that duo will take an awful lot out of you, don't fight.

Know yourself, know what you need, know your limits, and know what tomorrow will bring.

Drink wine like a snob

Here's what a true connoisseur does when faced with a good glass of wine: She sticks her nose way deep into the glass—as far as she can without the tip touching the liquid—breathes deeply, and inhales the scent. Then she does it again, swirling the wine and moving the glass around to extract as much nuance from the aroma as possible. This goes on for at least a minute or two while the connoisseur assesses the character and scents of the wine (called, in winespeak, the nose).

Once she's determined that she's got a nose of dried sour cherries steeped in rose hip tea, licorice, ink, attic dust, and something she can only describe as puppy breath, only then does she taste.

It is a tiny taste, a small sip that she rolls around her tongue and palate. She breathes in slightly while the liquid slides around her mouth so she can better discern flavors and mouthfeel. Then she swallows, having fully appreciated every last little aspect of said wine. At least three minutes have gone by.

Compare that to how fast the rest of us take a sip of wine.

OK, we're not saying you should drink every (or even any) glass of wine like our connoisseur friend. The point is, instead of just downing her glass of Sauvignon Blanc like so much cool water, she stops and considers. She acknowledges, appreciates, and makes the most of each sip.

And just as we strongly suggest you do with your steak fajita or Caesar salad, it's the same with drinking wine: Slow down. Enjoy. Focus. Not only will you probably end up drinking less than you usually do, you will appreciate it more.

And, ounce for ounce, wine has fewer calories than beer and straight liquor.

The Takeaway

- To slake thirst, make water (with or without bubbles and a squeeze of citrus) your go-to drink.

- Drinks with calories are like food. Don't let them slip down your throat without noticing.

- It's better (more nutritious, more filling) to eat fruit than drink fruit juice.

- Alcohol eats away at your ability to resist mindless nacho nibbling and more alcohol imbibing. When you're drinking, drink for fun, but drink responsibly (for a whole host of reasons, not just your waistline).

- When ordering a cocktail, think sophisticated, think simple.

- With fewer calories than beer or a fancy, fruity cocktail, wine is your friend. Sip it slowly, sniff, swirl, and savor it. You'll end up consuming less than you might of other tipples.

Chapter 11

The Balance Beam

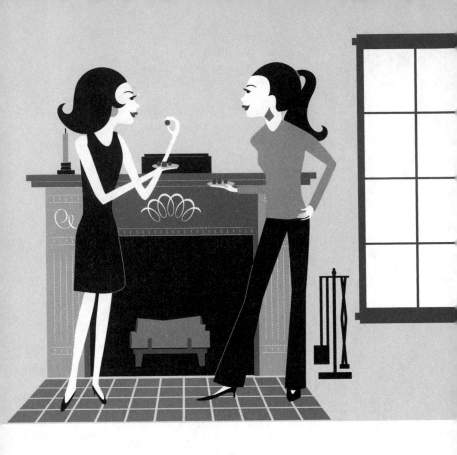

Get a little, give a little

Remember the Sigerson Morrison boots you fell in love with several chapters ago? And remember their price tag? It was probably more than you would typically spend on an impulse buy. Spending that much usually takes some thought because it's likely that once the money is spent, somewhere along the line you'd have to give something else up (that new silver handbag, tickets to a much-hyped show, the top-of-the-line cell phone).

If you've ever made this kind of bargain with your bank account, then you already know, on some level, exactly how to balance how much to eat in a day. If you buy something pricey (a pair of suede boots) during one credit card cycle or eat something rich (a hot fudge sundae) at one meal, go leaner the next time around.

We've told you before that you aren't good or bad for eating any particular food. You're not a sinner for diving into a slice of flourless chocolate cake and you're not a saint if you opt for fruit.

In both instances you're a person who has made a choice about what to eat.

It's all relative

Your food choices cannot be made in a vacuum. Throughout each day we need to evaluate our choices so our meals become a series of checks and balances. In other words, in order to eat what you want (without adding on the pounds), you must think about your meals and snacks in relation to one another. Before you order lunch, take 10 seconds to consider what you had for breakfast and what you will have for dinner.

This isn't a big deal. Approached with the right attitude—that is, a healthier choice after a less healthy one is not a punishment but a complement—it quickly becomes second nature. Think of it this way: You can have your cake and eat it too, but you can't have cake for lunch and conveniently forget about it at dinner.

Examples, please!

OK, it's time for some concrete advice. If for lunch you've chosen to eat a Reuben sandwich (either half or whole), you should have a piece of fruit or some carrot sticks for a snack, and for dinner maybe Quick Kale and White Bean Soup (page 199) or Caesar Salad to Die (But Not Get Fat) For (page 192).

If you had a huge sausage-and-omelet breakfast, you might not want much for lunch. Maybe you'll want a Quick Mushroom Salad with Aged Parmesan and Oregano (page 163) and a small whole grain roll with a little butter, if you like. Later for a snack you might have a small handful of nuts or some fruit and Roasted Tofu with Shiitake, Soy, and Ginger over Baby Spinach (page 197) for dinner. And maybe only half a cookie for dessert.

Or if you know you're going to pass by the exquisite gelato place later in the day (it's right next door to your hairdresser's, for goodness' sake!), don't deny yourself. Just plan the rest of your meals around that scoop of pistachio lusciousness.

This is not rocket science. Instituting a series of mental checks and balances allows you to eat what you want and gives you some guidance when you're not sure what exactly you want and therefore can't use desire as a guide.

The fresh and the cooked

Here's another way to think about balancing your meals and snacks. If the last thing you ate was fried, then the next thing you eat should be as fresh and raw or as lightly cooked as possible. (Think grilled, steamed, or sauteed with a scant amount of olive oil.) If you last ate something doughy and baked, then you should next eat something fresh and juicy (and not a frozen juice bar). And if the last thing you ate was processed, then the next thing you eat should definitely be fresh. And by "fresh" we mean fruits, vegetables, seeds, and nuts, not a freshly baked croissant.

Snack matters

We think snacks are very important, but you've got to be conscious of your snacking. Just because you were standing up while you ate that tiny handful of M&M's at your coworker's desk doesn't mean they should slip under the snack radar. Too often when we think about what we should have for dinner, we forget about those M&M's or the bag of chips we had while waiting in line at the grocery store. Forgetting about the snacks is especially dangerous around the holidays when (a) little cookies, cakes, and wrapped candies are everywhere and (b) you tend to go out to more big meals and buffets than usual. A little snack may be forgettable to you, but your little black dress remembers.

Holidays or not, be both strategic and conscious about snacking. Whether you're snacking for hunger or the yum factor, be strict about portions, especially if you're having something on the decadent side of the spectrum (a piece of rocky road fudge). Consider these *Skinny* tips for keeping snacking in the balance:

1. If you're craving something particular, a little bit of it can be extremely satisfying.

2. If you just want to eat to eat something, go for fresh fruit or vegetables.

3. A small handful of nuts (not honey-roasted) can go a long way because they have protein and fat. Plus, they're

BREAKING IT DOWN: A BAGEL BREAKFAST

Balancing food during the day can be tough, especially if you're not aware that you're eating more than you think. Consider the effect of a common breakfast—a poppy-seed bagel, shmear of cream cheese, and grande (medium) skinny latte—on the rest of your day.

The bagel: A bagel is the equivalent of about five slices of bread, and a slice of bread is one serving. Experts say you should eat somewhere between 4 and 11 grain servings a day. That's a pretty big spread, but the bottom line is that with one bagel you've already made vast inroads on the grains front.

Cream cheese: Experts recommend 0 to 3 servings of dairy a day. Even if you ate low-fat cream cheese, and even if you wiped some of it off your bagel (because it probably came with about a quarter pound of cream cheese), you can safely guess that you've had at least one serving of dairy.

The grande, skinny latte: Fat-free milk in the latte is a good choice. But along with the cream cheese on the bagel, you've used up your daily dairy allotment.

What does this breakfast mean for the rest of the day? You've already eaten a lot of grains and dairy, which has protein and saturated (bad) fat. But you haven't had any vegetables, fruit, lean protein (chicken, tofu, fish, beans), or good fats.

So on *The Skinny,* we'd recommend for lunch you have a green salad, very lightly dressed with olive oil, lemon, and salt. Toss in a cup of beans or a small (palm of your hand size) piece of grilled salmon, chicken, or tofu.

For a snack have a medium-size piece of fruit and/or a small handful of nuts. And for dinner have a pile of vegetables, a small portion (about 3 to 6 ounces) of protein, and half cup (cooked) of a whole grain such as barley, quinoa, brown rice, or whole wheat couscous. Dessert? Some fruit, such as two fresh figs and maybe a cookie.

For specifics on what to eat, see "2-Week Meal Plan," page 227.

good for you and taste great with a small handful of raisins or, you know, a little bit of chocolate.

4. Think of a banana as your go-to snack. Or try an apple (with or without a little bit of cheese), a pear, or some carrots (with or without some dip).

5. Snack ruts, if they're a fruit, veggie, or nut rut, are not all that bad. It's not like a chili cheese fries rut, after all.

Life in the balance: Does it ever end?

You may be thinking, "If eating all of the crème brûlée last night means I have to be careful all day today and maybe even skip the cookie I want now, how's that having what I want? Isn't that simply guilt of crèmes brûlées past?"

And the answer is: You decide how far is far enough. How far you need to take the checks and balances really comes down to what your goals are.

If you want to lose weight, you have to be more conservative (i.e., eat lean protein and greens for dinner if you want crème brûlée for dessert) than if you're in maintenance mode (when you can have more of the crème brûlée).

It also depends on what your attitude is. Does eating this way feel like a burden or is it liberating? We believe life on *The Skinny* is liberating because while decadent foods are limited, they're not forbidden.

You can choose to feel guilty or denied or indignant about having or not having your entire crème brûlée and your cookies at the same time. Or like us, you can feel happy about having some of that crème brûlée and having reveled in the moment when you were eating it. And you can feel all that and realize you'll have a cookie really soon. Not right away, but soon enough.

Prepping for the big night out

When you know a Very Big Meal is going to be part of your day, you have to prepare for it. Here are the three areas you need to think about:

- Exercise. (Do it the day of or the day after, depending on your schedule.)

- Outfit. (Choose one for the day of and the day after, if you're traveling. For the day after, choose something you feel swishy and sleek in but that isn't clingy.)

- Meals. (You know what we're going to say. Or wait, maybe not.)

For the meals leading up to the Big One, Melissa would skip and Robin would eat lightly but consistently throughout the day.

Robin would eat lightly for the classic reasons:

1. She'd rather poke her eyes out than miss a meal.

2. If Robin sat down to dinner after not eating since breakfast, extreme eating would ensue.

3. All that denial during the day would make Robin feel so indignant she would eat even more just to soothe her appetite's sense of being put on the back burner.

But for Melissa, skipping a meal is a reasonable and well-tried strategy when there's heavy eating on the horizon. Why?

1. She doesn't feel denied by not eating when she knows something great is around the corner.

2. She is extremely disciplined about her food.

3. She is conscientious about her nutritional needs and knows that missing one meal, for her, is not that big a deal.

All this to say, whatever path you choose when facing the feast—meal moderation or meal skipping—choose one tactic and stick to it. Every time. Christmas, Thanksgiving, Passover, Easter, July 4th, Boxing Day, Superbowl Sunday. Do not go blindly into that big meal.

MAKE THE "GOOD FOR YOU" GREAT

It's inevitable. We fall into the trap of thinking that really "great" foods are sticky buns and cheeseburgers. That "really great" and "good for you" must be mutually exclusive. But really great food is just really great food, be it fresh snow peas or ripe raspberries or snappy sauteed broccoli. Those are really great foods. Don't forget about them when you're hungry.

Sticking with The Skinny all day

You've decided to take our *Skinny* advice and balance your meals throughout the day. Now the question is, when is the best time to start? We say, right now, at your very next meal. No matter if you just finished an entire pint of frozen yogurt, half a bag of cookies, or an order of eggs Benedict.

ROBIN ON BAKING AND BALANCE

I like to bake. Not only do I love to eat the fruits of my labor (cookies, cakes, brownies), but I also like the process of baking itself.

Rather than give up baking on *The Skinny*, I've just made a few adjustments to my baking schedule. Here's what I do:

• Freeze it. The freezer is your friend. Pop in cookies, scones, and buttermilk biscuits, then take them out one at a time—and not one after the other one at a time. One a day per person at a time.

• Give it away. Did you bake a cake? Have a slice, save two slices. Give the rest away (to your neighbors, to anyone).

• Bake special. If you can't keep baked goods on hand, don't bake regular stuff. Plan a baking extravaganza when you'll make bread that will take all day, a tart with a persnickety crust and a homemade curd, or maybe cupcakes with fancy flowers on top. Work out all that baking love in one big, floured poof.

Starting and staying with *The Skinny* philosophy means that everything you choose to eat or not eat is just a choice. In other words, forgo thinking "I had an egg-on-a-roll with cheese and a full-fat latte for breakfast, so what the hell? I'll have a burger and fries for lunch and tempura for dinner. Tomorrow I'll go back on *The Skinny*."

That's not *The Skinny*. That's The Guilty. That's falling into the trap of thinking food is good or bad, and you are good or bad if you eat this or that, so you might as well start tomorrow when you'll have a clean slate.

But really, there's no "I'll be 'good' tomorrow" because there's no "good." There's no "bad." There's not even any tomorrow. There's just you about to eat your next meal, with another choice to make.

Because when you decide you're going to live with *The Skinny*'s system of checks and balances, you don't have to "give up" on any day. It's all about right now, what's next, and, most important, what you know in the long term will feel right for your body.

The Takeaway

- Think about the food you're about to eat in relation to the food you've had or will have during the day.

- Don't compare Milky Ways and watercress salads. Eat and enjoy each on its own terms.

- You can't be "good" tomorrow and "bad" today. You're just going to eat something in a couple of hours, so let it be tasty and preferably healthful, not guilty.

- If you know a big spread is on your schedule, don't pretend that it isn't.

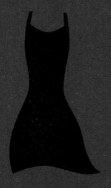

Emergency! The two-week LBD* plan

We've all been there—an event is two weeks away, and your standby LBD (*little black dress) would look even more fabulous without those extra five pounds. Well, guess what? You're in luck! *The Skinny* is to the rescue!

The first 5 to 10 pounds anyone loses on a diet is mostly water weight. It comes off fairly easily if you use a very disciplined approach. So if you haven't shed any pounds in a while, and you need to take them off fast, you can.

We won't promise the weight will stay off. No, that would take more patient weight loss and more sustained changes in habit. But for the big party in the little dress? You can do it, and that may inspire you to make more permanent lifestyle changes. Try not to binge at the party or in the days after. In fact, use the two-week countdown as your jump-start to new eating habits. And get ready for all the compliments your littler little black dress will inspire.

10 Skinny tips for quick weight loss

1. Exercise: You must do more. You must do cardio. Go for a brisk, 30-minute walk every night after dinner. If you're already working out three times a week, add a fourth or fifth 30-minute session to your regular routine, or add a challenging yoga class.

2. Less wine, fewer cocktails, no beer: As you know, we don't think life on *The Skinny* should be dry, but if you want to lose weight fast, cut out as much alcohol as you can during these two weeks. Stick to wine for whatever alcoholic drinks you have. And drink more water. Do. Not. Drink. Beer.

3. Farewell, lattes. You don't need us to tell you to switch to plain joe with just a little milk, do you?

4. Don't have the whole bagel. If you want a bagel, have half with a slice of yogurt cheese just once or twice during these two weeks. Poach any eggs you eat. Considering a muffin? Puh-lease. Next month. Not now. Make breakfast a cup of whole grain cereal with fat-free milk (or soymilk) and half a banana (have the second half later in the day as a snack). Or try a cup of fat-free, plain yogurt with half a banana and/or some strawberries or blueberries.

5. Snack on tea. Or eat some watermelon, an apple, or an orange. If you seriously crave a Danish and can limit yourself to two or three bites, have it. If you know you won't be able to stop at three bites, don't have any.

6. Space your food. Having a sandwich for lunch? Eat half at lunch with a salad or brothy soup and half later in the afternoon for a snack, along with a piece of fruit.

7. Portions, portions, portions. Keep them small. Don't eat too little, but eat very slowly and really think about whether you need more before you take seconds.

8. Do not eat fried or greasy foods. No french fries, grilled cheese, or onion rings. (If you can stop at one or two fries, have one or two, but in a LBD emergency we think it's easier to skip the fried thing entirely than to stop after a bite or two.) And no nachos. (You do want that little black dress to fit in two weeks, don't you?)

9. Keep your hands busy. After dinner, when you're watching TV or at a table where people are picking at food, keep your hands busy or sit on them. Bored hands nosh.

10. Evaluate. If you find that following these rules is making you miserable or you feel like Big Brother is watching every bite you take, say to hell with it. You'll look gorgeous no matter what you wear to that party. And if you still want to lose those 5 pounds, start snacking on fruit and slowly incorporating other *Skinny* changes into your diet.

The Skinny Recipes

Let's get cooking!

So that you may easily practice what we insistently preach throughout this book (in case you forgot, eat more fruits and vegetables), we offer you these produce-rich recipes. Each one is for a dish where a big serving of fruit and/or vegetables fills your plate and a smaller (4- to 6-ounce) serving of a protein (chicken, fish, meat, tofu) rounds out your meal.

These recipes are extremely simple, relatively quick, and, of course, completely delicious. They are exactly the kinds of dishes we love to eat and have the time to make on any given evening after work. They require very few ingredients—with one or two exceptions, you should be able to find all of them at your local supermarket. They require very little chopping. And on the nights when you can't bear to even lift a knife or turn on the stove, we've suggested ways to make a few of your favorite take-out standbys *Skinny*.

Recipe hints for Skinny girls

1. Anytime we call for butter in a savory dish, you can substitute olive oil. (Don't try this with sweets.)

2. We strongly recommend against using margarine or butter substitutes, which are typically full of trans fats. Some butter substitutes might not have trans fats, but they just won't give the same satisfying flavor as the real deal. So even if you just use a little, please use butter and/or olive oil.

3. If you're in weight losing mode (or maintenance mode, for that matter) and concerned about the amount of butter, oil, or sugar in a recipe, feel free to experiment with the amounts. No recipe is written in stone.

Stock up on Skinny staples

The first order of business when living on *The Skinny* is to head to the grocery store.

FOR THE PANTRY

Anchovies

Beans: chickpeas and/or white beans, canned

Broth/Bouillon: chicken, vegetable, beef

Capers

Chocolate (for eating and/or baking)

Crushed red pepper

Cumin

Extra virgin olive oil

Garlic

Honey

Nuts (almonds, cashews, pecans, walnuts, whatever)

Oatmeal (steel cut, whole grain)

Red wine vinegar

Rice wine vinegar

Roasted (Asian) **sesame oil**

Salt: (kosher or sea)

Soy sauce

Tapenade

Unbleached all-purpose flour

Whole wheat flour

FOR THE FREEZER

Blueberries/Strawberries/
Peaches/Raspberries
(or your favorite frozen fruit)

Broccoli

Boneless, skinless chicken
breast

Edamame

Peas

Shrimp

String Beans

FOR THE FRIDGE

Butter

Ginger

Olives

Onions

Yogurt

Tofu

The Skinny's weekly buys

Cheese: Pick something you like, and something different each week.

Fish/meat/chicken (4 to 6 ounces per person): Ask your butcher or fishmonger how long what you've bought should keep in the fridge.

Fruit: Get some bananas (if you like them) plus two or three different kinds of fruit, such as strawberries, apples, and a melon.

Salad greens: Select arugula, watercress, romaine, endive, or spring mix.

Fresh veggies: Pick three a week depending on what you think you'll make. We typically keep at least carrots, cucumbers, celery, and tomatoes on hand.

Herbs: Buy two fresh bunches per week. Usually you can substitute whatever you have on hand for what's in a recipe. We often keep basil, rosemary, and parsley in the fridge.

The fish list

So just what fish should you buy? An article in *The New York Times* suggested these:

WILD FISH

Anchovies

Arctic Char (color added)

Atlantic Butterfish

Black Cod (sable, Butterfish on West Coast)

Black Sea Bass

Haddock

Hake (white, silver, and red)

Hake (Chilean, Cape, and Argentine)

Halibut (Pacific only)

Herring

Mackerel (Atlantic or Boston only)

Mahi Mahi

Pacific Cod

Pacific Sand Dab (yellowtail flounder)

Pacific Whiting

Plaice

Porgy

Salmon (Pacific)

Sardines

Shad

Smelt

Sole (gray, petrale, rex, yellowfin)

Sole (Dover; English or lemon)

Whitefish

FARMED FISH

Carp

Catfish (domestic)

Striped Bass (rockfish)

Tilapia

Trout (rainbow, steelhead)

SHELLFISH

Clams (northern quahogs)

Clams (Atlantic surf, butter, Manila, ocean quahog, Pacific geoduck, Pacific littleneck and softshell)

Crab (Florida stone, Jonah, king)

Crayfish (United States)

Lobster (American)

Mussels (farmed blue, wild blue)

Mussels (New Zealand green, Mediterranean)

Oysters (farmed Eastern and Pacific)

Scallops (bay; Northeast, Canadian sea)

Shrimp (wild American pink, white, and brown)

Shrimp (spot prawns and northern shrimp)

Spiny Lobster (Caribbean, United States, and Australia)

Squid

Breakfast - The Foundation Meal

Whole Grain French Toast with Fresh Papaya

Use a soft whole grain loaf for this recipe—anything crusty or crunchy would distract from the smooth, custardy texture of the French toast. Papayas are an underappreciated fruit that deserve more play. We chose to pair them with this recipe because their juicy, bright flavor is a nice contrast to the fried bread, and, well, because we love them. But feel free to substitute whatever fruit you like.

Prep Time: 15 minutes **Makes:** 2 servings

1	medium papaya
½	cup milk
1	large egg
1	tablespoon sugar
½	teaspoon vanilla extract
	Pinch salt
4	slices whole grain bread (½ to ¾ inch thick)
½	tablespoon unsalted butter, plus additional, if necessary
	Maple syrup, for serving, optional

1. Peel the papaya and cut it in half lengthwise. Use a spoon to remove the seeds. Slice the papaya into cubes (you should have about 1 cup).

2. In a large shallow bowl whisk together the milk, egg, sugar, vanilla, and salt. Dip each slice of bread into the egg mixture, soaking both sides so that the bread is well coated and has absorbed the custard.

3. Melt the butter in a large pan over medium-high heat. Add the bread and cook, working in batches, if necessary, until golden brown, about 2 minutes per side. Add additional butter to the pan if the bread seems to be sticking.

4. Transfer the French toast to two serving plates and drizzle with maple syrup, if desired. Top with the chopped papaya and serve.

THE BIG HITS

Did you ever think you'd see a recipe for French toast in a book about keeping trim? But you know we're all about eating well. The best French toast is made with stale bread; use whole grain bread if possible because it's full of B vitamins, fiber, and iron and gives you some satisfying heft with which to start the day. The papaya gives you carotenes, vitamin C, the B vitamins folate and pantothenic acid, potassium, magnesium, and—as in all fruit—fiber.

Muesli with Raisins, Nuts, and Apple or Pear

This recipe is great to make in double or triple batches since it will keep in the refrigerator for up to one week. If you're using plain yogurt instead of vanilla, you may want to sweeten the muesli with a drizzle of honey or maple syrup. We like to eat this in the summertime in place of hot oatmeal.

Prep Time: 15 minutes, plus 15 minutes chilling   **Makes:** 4 servings

For the Muesli:

- 1   cup rolled oats
- ¼   cup golden raisins
- ¼   cup chopped dried apricots, figs, or prunes
- 2   tablespoons dried cranberries or cherries, optional
- 1½   cups plain or vanilla yogurt

For Each Serving:

- 1   small apple or firm pear such as Bosc
- 1   tablespoon chopped, toasted nuts, such as hazelnuts, walnuts, or almonds
   Honey or maple syrup, optional

1. In a medium bowl combine the oats, raisins, dried apricots, cranberries, and yogurt. Transfer the mixture to the refrigerator to chill for at least 15 minutes or up to a week.

2. Using a box grater, shred the apple, or finely chop the fruit with a knife.

3. To serve, spoon one-fourth of the muesli mixture into a bowl and stir in the shredded fruit. Garnish with toasted nuts and a drizzle of honey or maple syrup, if desired.

THE BIG HITS

When you have yogurt topped with granola, do you know what you're really eating? An oatmeal cookie. Most granola is full of honey and butter—that's not necessarily bad, but it's something to remember. So if granola is an oatmeal cookie, what's muesli? It's all the good whole grains that are in granola but without all the sweeteners and fat. Our version gives you fiber, B vitamins, and vitamin C. And when it comes to the honey or syrup, you get to decide how much to put in and how cookie-ish it'll be.

Whole Wheat Cherry Scones

The whole wheat flour makes these scones slightly more healthful than most and, we think, heartier and even more tasty. We love them split and topped with yogurt and strawberries for a shortcake stand-in that you could serve for breakfast, brunch, or even dessert if you sweeten the berries with a little honey or confectioner's sugar. Scones freeze really well too, so make the whole batch and keep the leftovers in a plastic bag in the freezer for an instant tea time treat.

Prep Time: 35 minutes   **Makes:** 12 scones

- ¾ cup dried cherries or cranberries, or raisins, very roughly chopped
- 2 cups all-purpose flour
- 1 cup whole wheat flour
- ¼ cup sugar
- 1 tablespoon baking powder
- 1 teaspoon ground cinnamon
- ½ teaspoon salt
- 5 tablespoons unsalted butter, cubed
- 2 large eggs
- ½ cup milk, plus additional for brushing

1. Preheat the oven to 450° F. Line a large baking sheet with parchment. Place the cherries in a sieve and pour boiling water over them. Transfer the cherries to a bowl and let cool.

2. In a large bowl combine the flours, sugar, baking powder, cinnamon, and salt.

3. Add the butter and, using a pastry cutter or a fork, cut the butter into the dry ingredients until the mixture resembles coarse crumbs. Stir in the cherries.

4. In a separate bowl whisk together the eggs and milk. Pour the liquid into the dry ingredients. Stir until the mixture just comes together (there should be no dry patches but do not overmix).

5. Divide the dough into three equal balls. With the palm of your hand, flatten each ball into a 5-inch disk. Using a knife, slice each disk into quarters. Transfer the scones to the prepared baking sheet, 1 to 2 inches apart. Brush each scone with additional milk.

6. Bake until the scones are golden on top and firm but not dry, 10 to 15 minutes. Let cool for 10 minutes before serving.

THE BIG HITS

Unless you've been living under a rock, you know that whole grains are *it*. Food companies are rolling out whole grain versions of all kinds of snacks, and bread makers everywhere are baking huskier versions of their loaves. These scones incorporate healthful whole grains, which give you fiber, iron, B vitamins, and more. You can make the scones in any size from tiny on up to satisfy your desire for a breakfast baked treat any time of day.

Maple Caramelized Apples

These caramelly apples are excellent mixed into yogurt, oatmeal, or as a topper for French toast (page 146) or peanut butter-smeared toast. Since the maple syrup adds plenty of sweetness here, it's best to use tart apples such as Granny Smith or Macoun for this recipe. By the way, try this with a sprinkle of sea salt at least once. It heightens the flavors and adds a salty zing that's a terrific contrast to the syrup—a little like chocolate-covered pretzels—without the chocolate or the pretzels.

Prep Time: 15 minutes **Makes:** 2 servings

- 3 tablespoons maple syrup
- 2 Granny Smith apples, peeled, cored, and cut into 8 wedges
- 2 teaspoons unsalted butter
  Ground cinnamon, optional
  Coarse sea salt, optional

1. Place a skillet large enough to hold the apples in a single layer over medium-high heat. Pour in the maple syrup and let simmer until slightly thickened, about 3 minutes.

2. Place the apples and the butter in the pan. Reduce the heat to low and cover the pan. Cook, turning and basting occasionally, until fork tender, 5 to 7 minutes.

3. Transfer the apples to serving plates and drizzle with the remaining syrup from the pan. Serve sprinkled with cinnamon and/or sea salt, if desired.

THE BIG HITS

This little dish has lots to offer in both flavor and nutrients. The maple syrup has potassium, and the apples have soluble and insoluble fiber, which helps prevent heart disease and keeps you "regular," plus vitamin C and other nutrients. But beyond all that, these apples are just so damned good, so easy to make, and a tiny bit decadent.

Retro Broiled Grapefruit

Remember diet books that preached the wonders of grapefruit for breakfast? We like it then or anytime. While a grapefruit is not quite enough for lunch, it does make a terrific sweet snack, especially if you add maple syrup, honey, or brown sugar.

If you don't have grapefruit spoons, you might want to separate the fruit into segments before topping and broiling. To do so, insert a paring or grapefruit knife between the grapefruit and its peel and run it around the fruit, loosening it from the peel. Then cut through the segments so they're easy to spoon out after the grapefruit's cooked.

Prep Time: 10 minutes **Makes:** 2 servings

- 1 grapefruit (pink, white, or ruby, as you wish)
- 1 to 1½ tablespoons maple syrup, honey, or brown sugar
- 2 teaspoons butter

1. Preheat the broiler.

2. Halve the grapefruit and place it cut sides up on a broiler-safe baking dish. Top each half with half the sweetener of choice and a teaspoon of butter cut into tiny bits and scattered over the surface of the grapefruit.

3. Broil for 3 to 4 minutes, until the butter is melted and the grapefruit is warmed through. Serve warm.

THE BIG HITS

A grapefruit's biggest nutritional hit is from vitamin C, which is an antioxidant that can help reduce "free radicals." Free radicals are unstable molecules that attack other molecules and cause oxidation, which damages cells; rust is an example of oxidation—outside your body, of course. Half of a grapefruit also has 2 grams of fiber. Current recommendations are for adults to eat 25 to 30 grams of fiber per day, but most Americans only eat 14 to 15 grams in a day. So every bit of fiber you squeeze into your daily meals is a good thing.

Ginger-Stewed Rhubarb with Yogurt

Soft, tart stewed rhubarb, spiced up with fresh ginger and served with creamy yogurt, makes an excellent breakfast or snack. We suggest using full-fat or low-fat yogurt here, rather than nonfat. Most nonfat brands are too acidic to work well with rhubarb. Thick and tangy Greek yogurt is hands down our favorite. Feel free to double or triple the recipe. The rhubarb compote will keep for at least a week or two in the fridge.

Prep Time: 20 minutes   **Makes:** 2 servings

- ¼ cup light brown sugar
- 1 (1-inch) piece fresh ginger, grated
- 8 ounces rhubarb, trimmed and cut into 1-inch pieces (about 1½ cups)
- 2 cups Greek, plain, or vanilla yogurt, for serving

1. In a medium pot over medium-high heat bring the sugar, ginger, and 2 tablespoons water to a boil. Cook until the sugar dissolves completely, about 5 minutes.

2. Stir in the rhubarb and reduce the heat to low. Simmer, covered, until the rhubarb is completely tender and falling apart, about 10 minutes.

3. Spoon the yogurt into two bowls and top with the compote.

THE BIG HITS

Here's the good news: Rhubarb has calcium. Here's the bad news: Like spinach, rhubarb has something called oxalic acid, which makes the calcium hard for the body to absorb. But here's other good news: Rhubarb's got vitamin C too, and it has a lot of fiber—in fact, rhubarb was once used as a laxative. Its nutrients are antioxidizing, boost your immune system, aid in digestion, and help fight heart disease.

Almond Butter and Strawberry Breakfast Smoothie

This is so good it could practically be dessert. You know how we feel about dessert for breakfast. But really, it's too healthful to be sinful. While almond butter goes really well with the strawberries, peanut butter will work well too. Fresh strawberries are always tasty, but use the same amount of frozen strawberries if you have them on hand.

Prep Time: 5 minutes **Makes:** 2 servings

- 1 pint strawberries, hulled
- 1 cup plain soymilk, plus additional if necessary
- 2 tablespoons almond butter
- 2 teaspoons honey

1. Combine all of the ingredients in a blender and puree until smooth. Thin out with additional soymilk to reach desired consistency.

THE BIG HITS

Strawberries have loads of fiber and vitamin C—ounce for ounce, more than citrus fruits. In an analysis done by the USDA, strawberries come in second only to the famous blueberry in antioxidants. (Vitamin C is an antioxidant.) The downside of strawberries is that when grown conventionally, as most are, they carry a high pesticide load. So wash them well by soaking them for 10 minutes (some say add a tiny touch of soap; others say don't bother) and then rinsing them. If possible, buy fresh or frozen organic berries.

Banana and Kiwi Smoothie

When what we really want for breakfast is cookies, sometimes we double the maple syrup in this recipe. But on more normal days, we like this au naturel, without any sweetening, letting the fruity flavors of the kiwi and bananas shine. If you hate or don't have kiwis on hand, you can substitute ½ cup of other fruits, such as berries, peaches, or plums.

Prep Time: 5 minutes **Makes:** 2 servings

- 1 banana, peeled and cut into chunks
- 1 kiwifruit, peeled and sliced (about ½ cup)
- 1 cup low-fat yogurt
- ½ cup ice cubes
- 2 teaspoons or even a little more maple syrup, optional

1. Combine all of the banana, kiwi, yogurt, ice, and syrup in a blender and whir together until smooth. Pour into glasses and serve immediately.

THE BIG HITS

This is simple. Bananas have potassium. Studies have shown that potassium-rich foods lower blood pressure. (So if you can't get to the gym to blow off steam after a bad day, have a banana.) Bananas also have fiber, which reduces the risk of heart disease, diabetes, and, you know, constipation. (We'd whisper that if we could.) Here's another bit of (sort of) good news: Both the banana and kiwi consistently rank among the fruits and veggies least contaminated by pesticides (see page 87 for a list of the most- and least-contaminated produce).

Lunch

Perfect Green Salad with Grainy Mustard Dressing

This is the vinaigrette to keep in the fridge for whenever the salad urge strikes. You can double, triple, or multiply the recipe ad infinitum depending upon how much salad you eat. It will keep for at least a week.

Prep Time: 5 minutes   **Makes:** 2 to 4 servings

1½   quarts washed salad greens

For the Vinaigrette:

1   tablespoon red wine vinegar
1   teaspoon grainy Dijon mustard
½   teaspoon finely chopped garlic
3   tablespoons extra virgin olive oil
Coarse sea salt or kosher salt and freshly ground black pepper

1. To make the vinaigrette, whisk together the vinegar, mustard, and garlic in a small bowl.

2. Pour in the oil in a slow, steady stream, whisking constantly until incorporated.

3. Place the salad greens in a large bowl. Add enough of the dressing to coat the greens evenly and toss the salad gently to combine. Season with salt and pepper to taste.

THE BIG HITS

Salad greens obviously rank high among our favorite go-to foods. With greens, we're not only getting a high-volume, low-calorie food, we're getting folate, fiber, vitamin C, and depending on how green the greens are, some beta-carotene (so we feel full, light, and quite antioxidized). This salad dressing also offers the heart-healthy, cholesterol-reducing benefits of raw garlic.

Instant Tricolor Salad with Olive Oil and Parmesan

The greatest thing about endive and radicchio is how easy they are to prepare. Just rinse, thinly slice, and watch the tight, coiled heads fall apart into colorful strands. When you mix them with bagged baby arugula, a little cheese, and some good olive oil, you don't even need a vinaigrette to produce a company-worthy salad in about 5 minutes flat.

Prep Time: 5 minutes   **Makes:** 2 to 4 servings

- 1   small head endive
- ½   head radicchio, halved and cored
- ½   ounce grated Parmesan cheese (about 2 tablespoons)
- 1   cup baby arugula, washed and dried
- 1   tablespoon extra virgin olive oil
- Coarse sea salt or kosher salt

1. Discard the outer browned leaves of the endive, rinse the bulb, and thinly slice crosswise into rounds. Rinse and slice the radicchio crosswise into thin half-moon shreds.

2. Place the endive and radicchio in a bowl, add the Parmesan, and toss to combine.

3. Divide the arugula among serving plates and top with the endive mixture. Drizzle with the olive oil and season with salt.

THE BIG HITS

Both endive and radicchio are a kind of chicory, which has been cultivated for centuries for its medicinal properties. Egyptians, Greeks, and Romans all considered chicory to be a blood and liver tonic. We know now that chicory has fiber, beta-carotene (an antioxidant), and potassium, among other nutrients. All contribute to long-term heart health and general wellness.

Greek Salad with Feta, Cucumbers, and Olives

Along with tomato and onion sandwiches on whole wheat toast, Greek salads are one of our favorite standbys when we're out at a diner. Our homemade version is much fresher and tastier. Soaking the feta takes out some of the salt, but that's strictly optional.

Prep Time: 20 minutes   **Makes:** 2 servings

- ¼   cup thinly sliced red onion
- 1   tablespoon, plus 2 teaspoons red wine vinegar
- 2   tablespoons extra virgin olive oil
- 1   teaspoon dried oregano, crumbled
- 1   head romaine, outer leaves discarded, trimmed, and cut into bite-size pieces (about 9 cups chopped)
- ¼   English cucumber, peeled, halved, and cut into ¼-inch-thick moons (about ½ cup sliced)
- ¾   cup cherry tomatoes, halved lengthwise (about ½ cup sliced)
- ⅓   cup thinly sliced, pitted kalamata olives
- 2   to 3 ounces feta cheese, to taste, soaked in water, drained, and crumbled (about ½ to ¾ cup)

    Coarse sea salt or kosher salt and freshly ground black pepper

1. In a small bowl combine the onion and 1 tablespoon of vinegar. Let soak for 10 minutes, then drain vinegar. (This will help cut the sharpness of the onion.) In a separate bowl whisk together the olive oil, remaining 2 teaspoons vinegar, and oregano.

2. In a large bowl combine the romaine, cucumber, tomatoes, olives, and red onion. Add the vinaigrette and toss gently to combine.

3. Sprinkle the crumbled feta on top of the salad and season to taste with salt and pepper. Toss again and serve.

THE BIG HITS

Let's talk about onions. Raw or cooked, they're very, very good for you. Onions have sulfur compounds that can help lower bad (LDL) cholesterol levels. They have flavonoids (anitoxidants found in plant pigments) that are anti-inflammatory and may help protect the lungs against cancer and asthma. They have other flavonoids that are antibacterial and protect the stomach from ulcers. And they've got fiber, vitamin C, folate, potassium, and calcium. When it comes to your health, onions are definitely worth any investment in breath mints that they require.

LUNCH

Pear, Watercress, and Blue Cheese Salad

This yummy salad is sophisticated and satisfying. It is crunchy from the watercress, salty and creamy from the blue cheese, and a little sweet from the pear. Of course, if you're not a blue cheese fan, sub in your favorite cheese.

Prep Time: 15 minutes **Makes:** 2 to 4 servings

- 1 tablespoon extra virgin olive oil
- ½ tablespoon freshly squeezed lemon juice
  Kosher salt and freshly ground black pepper
- 1 bunch watercress, stemmed
- 1 pear, cored and thinly sliced
- 1 to 2 ounces blue cheese, crumbled (about ¼ to ½ cup)

1. In a small bowl whisk together the olive oil and lemon juice and season with salt and pepper.

2. In a medium bowl combine the watercress and pear. Drizzle with the dressing and toss gently to combine.

3. Add the blue cheese and toss again to combine. Adjust seasoning, if necessary.

THE BIG HITS

Dark, leafy greens such as watercress contain folate, beta-carotene, and even calcium. Watercress also has some fluid-balancing potassium. And it tastes great, especially paired with a fiber- and vitamin C-rich pear.

Citrus Salad with Fennel, Olives, and Onions

The combination of juicy orange, savory olives, and crunchy fennel in this tasty winter salad makes it the ideal antidote to those times when you just can't face another lunch of tossed baby lettuces. If you don't have fennel, leave it out, or substitute 1 sliced endive or 1 peeled, seeded, and thinly sliced cucumber.

Prep Time: 15 minutes   **Makes:** 2 servings

- 2   oranges or 1 grapefruit
- 2   tablespoons extra virgin olive oil
-     Coarse sea or kosher salt and freshly ground black pepper
- 1   small fennel bulb
- ½   small sweet Vidalia or Walla Walla onion
- ¼   cup chopped pitted kalamata olives

1. Peel and segment the fruit (or peel it and slice it into wheels) and lay it out on a serving platter or divide it between two plates. Season with 1 tablespoon of the olive oil and salt and pepper to taste.

2. Trim off the fennel fronds and reserve them. Cut the base of the fennel bulb off and slip off the outer fennel layers (they are tough, and they will fall right off when you cut the bottom off the fennel). Halve the fennel lengthwise and thinly slice each half into half-moons. Scatter those over the citrus. Chop a tablespoon of the fennel fronds.

3. Thinly slice the onion and scatter over the fennel. Sprinkle the olives and chopped fennel fronds over all, drizzle with the remaining tablespoon of olive oil, and season with more salt and pepper.

THE BIG HITS

Oranges, grapefruit, and fennel serve up fiber and vitamin C—the latter chips away at those oxidizing free radicals that damage your cells. Fennel has potassium too, which will keep your fluids in balance, your nerve impulses shooting straight, and your blood pressure low. The olives are an excellent source of monounsaturated (good) fat. It lowers bad (LDL) cholesterol and helps raise good (HDL) cholesterol. And onions have sulfur compounds that are quite good for your heart.

Granny Smith Apple Salad with Cheddar

This is our version of a ploughman's lunch, which is a British tradition composed of apples, a hunk of cheese, and a loaf of bread (and usually a pint of beer). We've put it together (sans the pint) in a crunchy salad that's a little rich from the cheese and pleasantly tart from the apple and lemon juice. Aged cheddar (anything over a year old) has a drier, crumbly texture and more intense flavor, and works really well here. Or substitute your favorite cheese. Crumbled blue, always one of our picks, would be terrific.

Prep Time: 15 minutes   **Makes:** 2 servings (2 cups)

- 2   teaspoons extra virgin olive oil
- 1½   teaspoons freshly squeezed lemon juice
- 1   Granny Smith apple, quartered, cored, and thinly sliced
- ½   ounce sharp cheddar cheese, preferably aged (about 2 tablespoons)
  Coarse sea salt or kosher salt and freshly ground black pepper
- 2   tablespoons chopped fresh parsley, optional

1. In a medium bowl whisk together the olive oil and lemon juice.

2. Add the apple slices and toss to combine.

3. With a vegetable peeler, shave thin slices of cheddar into the salad. Add the salt, pepper, and parsley, if using. Gently toss the salad again, and serve.

THE BIG HITS

Apples have soluble and insoluble fiber, and because even a cut-up apple requires some real biting on your part, it cleans your teeth and stimulates your gums. The olive oil gives you some monounsaturated fat, which helps your cells work and lowers your bad cholesterol levels. The cheese offers a nice serving of calcium and protein.

...∧ Bean Salad with Basil and ...d-Boiled Egg

...is salad only gets better as it sits, so go ahead and make it the day before you want to serve it. Keep it in the fridge, then bring it to room temperature 20 minutes before you want to eat. The egg turns a bit brown from the balsamic in the dressing, but the flavors get deeper and richer as everything melds. Double this recipe to feed a crowd. It's terrific for a buffet or picnic because the beans won't wilt at room temperature.

Prep Time: 15 minutes   **Makes:** 2 servings

- 8   ounces green beans, trimmed
- 1   hard-boiled egg, peeled and roughly chopped (see note)
- 1   tablespoon chopped fresh basil
- 1   tablespoon extra virgin olive oil
- 2   teaspoons balsamic vinegar
-     Kosher salt and freshly ground black pepper

1. Fill a medium pot halfway with water and bring to a boil over medium-high heat. Add the beans and cook until crisp yet tender, 1 to 2 minutes. Drain and rinse under cold water to stop the cooking. Transfer the beans to a bowl.

2. Add the egg and basil to the beans. In a small bowl whisk together the oil and vinegar. Add the mixture to the beans and toss to combine. Season to taste with salt and pepper and serve.

Note: There are many ways to hard-boil an egg. Our favorite is to bring the egg(s) to a boil starting with cold water, letting it boil for a minute, then covering the pot and turning off the heat. Fifteen minutes or so later, the egg will be cool enough to peel and perfectly cooked.

THE BIG HITS

Green beans are chockfull of vitamin K, which is an antioxidant that helps blood clot and protects against osteoporosis by helping the body absorb calcium. They also have vitamins C and A, fiber, beta-carotene, folate, and iron. As for the egg, it has about 6 grams of protein, minerals such as iodine and zinc, and some vitamins. In other words, unless you really have a problem with cholesterol, an egg is a nutritional and filling food choice.

...ry Salad with Blue Cheese ...d Tabasco

If you ask us, the garnishes are the best part of eating Buffalo chicken wings. Not to say we don't also love the wings, but the combination of the cool, crisp celery, creamy blue cheese dressing, and the spiciness from the Tabasco is so addictive, we wanted to figure out a way to savor it more than every now and then. This recipe does the trick. It's excellent on its own but also makes a terrific accompaniment to grilled steak, salmon, and, of course, chicken.

Prep Time: 15 minutes   **Makes:** 2 servings

- ⅓ cup plain yogurt
- 1 teaspoon extra virgin olive oil
  Kosher salt and freshly ground black pepper
- 1 ounce blue cheese, crumbled (about ¼ cup)
- 3 stalks celery, trimmed and thinly sliced crosswise
  Tabasco sauce

1. In a large bowl whisk together the yogurt, oil, salt, and pepper. Fold in the blue cheese.

2. Add the celery and toss to combine. Top with several dashes of Tabasco sauce, to taste, and serve.

THE BIG HITS

Celery is more than just a dieter's fallback food. It has vitamin C (an antioxidant) and active compounds called pthalides that help lower blood pressure (a function long recognized in Chinese medicine). Celery is high in the minerals potassium and sodium, so it helps balance the body's fluids, acting as a diuretic.

Quick Mushroom Salad with Aged Parmesan and Oregano

Many supermarkets sell sliced, cleaned mushrooms that transform this from a quick salad to an instant one. Blue cheese is a great substitute for the Parmesan cheese.

Prep Time: 10 minutes   **Makes:** 1 serving

- 4 ounces white mushrooms, cleaned, trimmed, and sliced (about 1½ cups sliced)
- 1½ tablespoons extra virgin olive oil
- 2 teaspoons balsamic vinegar, plus additional to taste
- ¼ teaspoon crushed dried oregano
  Kosher salt and freshly ground black pepper
- ½ ounce aged Parmesan cheese (about 2 tablespoons)

1. Trim the stem ends of the mushrooms and slice the mushrooms into ¼-inch slices.

2. In a medium bowl, combine the mushrooms, oil, vinegar, oregano, and salt and pepper to taste. Toss well.

3. Using a vegetable peeler, peel the cheese into curls and mix gently into the salad. Taste and adjust the seasoning, if necessary, then serve.

THE BIG HITS

Mushrooms have selenium, a mineral that works with vitamin E to produce antioxidants and support the immune system and thyroid. Mushrooms also have potassium, which helps your heart stay in its normal rhythm and keeps your fluids in balance. Plus, they have riboflavin, which keeps your skin healthy and your vision sharp.

LUNCH

Tomato-Herb Salad with Goat Cheese

Tomatoes and goat cheese became a cliché in the 1980s, when chefs started putting goat cheese on everything. But we don't care. The mix of tart, creamy goat cheese and ripe, sweet-tart tomatoes flavored with plenty of herbs is a keeper. If you're not a goat cheese fan, you can substitute your favorite cheese here. Blue and feta are also traditional with tomatoes, while cheddar, Gruyère, and Brie are less expected, but no less compelling.

Prep Time: 15 minutes **Makes:** 2 servings

- 2 cups diced ripe tomatoes or halved cherry tomatoes
- 1 cup mixed fresh herb leaves, such as basil, parsley, mint, celery leaves, and lovage (use at least $\frac{1}{2}$ cup parsley)
- 2 ounces goat cheese, crumbled or cut into bits (about $\frac{1}{2}$ cup)
- $\frac{1}{4}$ teaspoon minced garlic
- $\frac{1}{8}$ teaspoon coarse sea or kosher salt, plus additional to taste
- 1 tablespoon extra virgin olive oil
  Freshly ground black pepper

1. In a medium bowl toss together the tomatoes, herbs, and goat cheese.

2. Using the flat side of a knife or a mortar and pestle, mash together the garlic and sea salt to form a paste. Transfer to a small bowl and stir in the olive oil. Pour the garlic oil into the salad and toss to combine. Add pepper and additional salt, if desired.

THE BIG HITS

Fiber, antioxidants, and vitamin C are just some of the benefits that come from tomatoes. Of course, this salad also gives you the heart-smart benefits of raw garlic (from its sulfur compounds) and olive oil (from its monounsaturated fats). And then there's the cheese. Goat cheese has just 60 calories and 5 grams of fat per ounce, compared to 100 calories and 10 grams of fat for an ounce of cream cheese. Plus, it has twice the amount of protein of cream cheese.

Roasted Asparagus with Herbs and Capers

Roasting vegetables might be our favorite way of preparing them. Not only is it incredibly easy (lightly rub the vegetable in question with olive oil, roast at high heat until softened and golden), the roasting adds a layer of caramelized flavor. Once you've had asparagus prepared this way, it's hard to go back to steamed.

Prep Time: 15 to 20 minutes **Makes:** 2 servings

- 1 pound asparagus, trimmed
- 1 tablespoon extra virgin olive oil
- Coarse sea salt or kosher salt and freshly ground black pepper
- 2 tablespoons chopped fresh herbs, such as a mix of basil, tarragon, and parsley (or all basil or all parsley)
- 2 teaspoons drained capers, chopped

1. Preheat the oven to 450°F.

2. In a bowl toss the asparagus with the olive oil and season lightly with salt and pepper.

3. Spread the asparagus in one layer on a baking sheet. Roast until just tender, 10 to 12 minutes, depending on the thickness of the asparagus (thinner ones will cook more quickly).

4. Transfer the asparagus to a serving dish and toss with the herbs and capers. Taste and adjust the seasoning, if necessary. Serve warm or at room temperature.

THE BIG HITS

Asparagus is full of the antioxidant vitamin K, which catches free radicals and helps the body absorb calcium. It also has vitamin C and folate, which is especially good for your heart. If you're thinking about becoming pregnant, eat a lot of folate because it supports healthy cell division in the nervous system of a fetus. If that weren't enough, asparagus has potassium and acts as a natural diuretic. Never mind that it makes urine smell a little funky; it's a small price to pay.

Pan-Seared Brussels Sprouts

Ahh, the magic of high heat. Searing Brussels sprouts over a high flame caramelizes them, changing their intense, slightly funky cabbagey flavor into a pure, sweet toastiness that we adore. Good hot or at room temperature, they also make a marvelous Thanksgiving side dish—probably the skinniest one on the table.

Prep Time: 15 minutes **Makes:** 2 to 4 servings

- 12 ounces Brussels sprouts (about 2 cups)
- 1 tablespoon extra virgin olive oil
  Coarse sea salt or kosher salt and freshly ground black pepper
  Lemon wedges, for serving

1. Trim the stem ends of the Brussels sprouts and cut them in half lengthwise.

2. Heat the oil in a medium skillet over high heat. Add the Brussels sprouts cut sides down and sear until they just begin to color, about 1 minute. Do not turn the sprouts.

3. Sprinkle the sprouts with salt and pepper. Reduce the heat to medium and cover the pan. Continue to cook the sprouts until tender, 7 to 10 minutes. Serve with lemon wedges.

THE BIG HITS

Brussels sprouts are a cruciferous vegetable like broccoli, cauliflower, and cabbage. Cruciferous vegetables contain a phytochemical called sulforaphane, which may help prevent cancer because it aids the liver in producing enzymes that detoxify cancer-causing agents. Cruciferous vegetables also have loads of vitamins and nutrients (folate, fiber, and vitamin C, to name a few) and when cooked correctly taste really good.

Toasted Broccoli with Cheddar

This is a skinny version of Welsh rarebit, with broccoli standing in for the bread. It's filling and fairly decadent in the amount of cheese we've used, but the broccoli balances the indulgence. If you want it even skinnier, use half the amount of cheese. Either way it's a terrific winter lunch.

Prep Time: 25 minutes   **Makes:** 1 to 2 servings

- 1 head broccoli (about 1½ pounds)
- 1 tablespoon extra virgin olive oil
- 2 ounces cheddar cheese, grated (about ½ cup)
  Coarse sea salt or kosher salt and freshly ground pepper

1. Preheat the oven to 400°F.

2. With a sharp knife, slice the broccoli from the stem into bite-size florets. Toss the broccoli with the olive oil and spread in a single layer on a baking sheet.

3. Bake for 10 minutes, then sprinkle evenly with the grated cheese. Return the broccoli to the oven and continue to roast until the broccoli is tender and the cheese is bubbling and golden, about 10 minutes more. Season with salt and pepper before serving.

THE BIG HITS

Love it or hate it (and we love it), broccoli is really good for you. (By the way, if you hate broccoli, don't eat it—nothing is so good for you that it warrants eating through distaste.) Broccoli has vitamins C, K, and A. It has folate to help produce and maintain cells and potassium to help balance fluid in the body. It's also very high in fiber. All this means it's good for your heart, your digestive system, your muscle function, your nerve endings, even your vision. So if you like broccoli, eat a lot of it.

Cucumber Yogurt Dill Soup

We love the instant gratification of blender soups, especially chilled, creamy, garlicky soups such as this one. If you're not a dill fan, this tastes equally excellent with basil.

Prep Time: 10 minutes   **Makes:** 2 servings

- 1   English cucumber, trimmed and cut into chunks
- 2   cups plain low-fat yogurt
- 1   garlic clove, chopped
- 1   tablespoon chopped fresh dill, plus additional for garnish
- 1½   teaspoons freshly squeezed lemon juice
- ½   teaspoon coarse sea salt or kosher salt
    Freshly ground black pepper

1. Place the cucumber, yogurt, garlic, dill, lemon juice, salt, and pepper in a blender or food processor and puree. If the mixture seems too thick, add a little water and blend to the desired consistency. Transfer the soup to the refrigerator and chill at least 20 minutes before serving. Garnish with fresh dill.

THE BIG HITS

Yogurt contains calcium, protein, and B vitamins. The culturing process that turns milk into yogurt also turns milk's lactose into lactic acid, making it potentially more tolerable to people whose stomachs are irritated by lactose. Look for yogurt that has "active yogurt cultures," "living yogurt cultures," lactobacillus, or acidophilus. These are the "good bacteria" that should be living in your intestines at all times.

Brown Bagging It— Yes, You Can Take It With You

Tuna and Cucumber Salad with Olives

For a real treat try this salad using leftover cooked fresh tuna or salmon in place of the canned.

Prep Time: 10 minutes **Makes:** 2 servings

- 1 tablespoon freshly squeezed lemon juice
- 1 tablespoon extra virgin olive oil
- 1 cup cubed cucumber
- 1 (6-ounce) can water-packed tuna, drained
- ¼ cup chopped, pitted kalamata olives
- 1½ tablespoons chopped scallion
- 1 tablespoon chopped fresh parsley
  Coarse sea salt or kosher salt and freshly ground black pepper

1. In a medium bowl whisk together the lemon juice and olive oil.

2. Add the cucumber, tuna, olives, scallion, and parsley and toss well. Season to taste with salt and pepper and serve.

Brown bag it with: a whole grain roll and a pear

THE BIG HITS

This recipe is a new take on an old favorite. By saying "so long" to mayo and "hello" to olive oil, you turn a heart-soggy dish into a heart-healthy one. The olives themselves give you even more good, filling fat that reduces bad cholesterol. And the cucumber is full of vitamin C. As for the tuna, it's a good source of lean protein and it has omega-3 essential fatty acids. If you're using canned tuna, choose light rather than white or albacore; light tuna has lower mercury levels because it comes from smaller fish, and smaller fish have less mercury stored in their fat.

Chicken Salad with Roasted Red Peppers

Dressed with roasted red peppers, olive oil, mustard, and garlic instead of the usual bland mayonnaise, this chicken salad packs a punch. It's great made into a sandwich for lunch at the office. Or if bread isn't on your menu, serve the chicken salad on a bed of greens tossed with a little olive oil and sprinkled with salt.

Prep Time: 15 minutes   **Makes:** 4 servings

- 2 teaspoons Dijon mustard
- 1 teaspoon white wine or sherry vinegar
- ½ garlic clove, minced
- 2 tablespoons extra virgin olive oil, plus extra, if desired
- ½ roasted chicken, skinned, meat removed from the bone, and roughly chopped (about 1½ cups meat)
- 1 stalk celery, chopped
- 3 tablespoons chopped roasted red bell peppers
- 1 tablespoon chopped chives
  Coarse sea salt or kosher salt and freshly ground black pepper
  Whole wheat bread or crusty white bread, for serving, optional
  Mixed salad greens, for serving, optional

1. To make the vinaigrette, in a small bowl whisk together the mustard, vinegar, and garlic. Whisking constantly, slowly add the olive oil until fully incorporated.

2. In a medium bowl combine the chicken, celery, red peppers, and chives. Fold in the vinaigrette. Season with salt and black pepper and serve, either made into a sandwich or over salad greens tossed with a little more olive oil and sprinkled with salt.

Brown bag it with: grapes

THE BIG HITS

The individual ingredients in this salad all have something to offer: The red bell peppers have vitamin C, beta-carotene, vitamin B_6, and fiber; the olive oil is a good monounsaturated fat; and skinless chicken, especially the white breast meat, is a good source of lean protein. But the real value in this salad is its style. By using oil instead of mayonnaise and a colorful veggie such as red peppers, you are taking an old-fashioned favorite and morphing it into a colorful, flavorful, and sophisticated dish (and, oh yes, healthful too).

Moroccan Carrot Salad with Coriander and Cashews

Harissa, a thick, pungent Moroccan hot sauce sold in tubes, gives this colorful salad its particular verve. If you can't find it (in gourmet specialty shops or a large supermarket), just substitute Tabasco, use pecans or peanuts in place of cashews, and change the name of the dish to Cajun Carrot Salad. Either way, the combination of chile sauce, carrots, and nuts is unusual and exceptionally delicious.

Prep Time: 15 minutes   **Makes:** 2 to 4 servings

- 1 pound carrots, peeled and trimmed
- 1/2 cup roasted cashews, roughly chopped
- 1/4 cup chopped fresh cilantro
- 1 tablespoon extra virgin olive oil
- 1 1/2 teaspoons freshly squeezed lemon juice
- 1/2 teaspoon harissa, plus additional, to taste, or Tabasco sauce, to taste
- 1/4 teaspoon ground coriander
- Coarse sea salt or kosher salt and freshly ground black pepper

1. Shred the carrots using a box grater or a food processor fitted with the grating attachment. Transfer the carrots to a bowl and add the cashews and cilantro.

2. In a small bowl whisk together the oil, lemon juice, harissa, and ground coriander. Pour the mixture over the carrots and toss to combine, seasoning with salt and pepper. Serve.

Brown bag it with: whole wheat pita and figs

THE BIG HITS

It's true what your mom used to say about carrots: They are good for your eyes. Their beta-carotene converts to vitamin A, which is what helps your night vision. Carrots also may help prevent lung cancer. Nuts, in general, are extremely nutritious. Cashews, in particular, have the good fat (like the stuff in olive oil) that lowers bad cholesterol. They also have magnesium, which helps keep bones strong and supports the smooth functioning of nerves and muscles.

Cabbage Roll-Ups with Gruyère, Mustard, and Caraway

We were hesitant when a (skinny) girlfriend told us about this veggie roll-up recipe, but since we tend to like anything with cheese, we gave this hard-to-define dish a try. We think of these as low-carb cheese wraps with cabbage leaves standing in for the usual flour tortilla or lavash bread or whatever else wraps a wrap. The mustard and caraway add a lot of flavor, and the cabbage makes for a nice and crunchy contrast. It's an unexpected winner!

Prep Time: 15 minutes   **Makes:** 1 serving (about 6 rolls)

- 1 head napa cabbage
- 1 ounce Gruyère cheese (about ¼ cup)
- 1 tablespoon Dijon mustard
- 1½ tablespoons mayonnaise
  Pinch caraway or cumin seeds

1. Remove the outer layers of the cabbage until you come to the pale, tender leaves beneath. Tear off 6 large, whole leaves. With a sharp knife completely slice the leaf from each side of the stem so that you have two leaf halves.

2. Using a cheese slicer or sharp knife, thinly slice the cheese. In a small bowl whisk together the mustard, mayonnaise, and caraway seeds.

3. Arrange the cabbage layers on a clean surface, overlapping two halves per roll. Brush each roll with some of the Dijon mixture. Divide the cheese slices among the 6 rolls.

4. Starting at the bottom of each set of leaves, roll the stuffed cabbage away from you. Tuck the loose end underneath the roll to secure. Serve.

Brown bag it with: breadsticks and clementines

THE BIG HITS

Napa cabbage, sometimes called Chinese cabbage, is part of the brassica family of vegetables. In addition to a boatload of vitamin C and fiber, brassica vegetables have phytonutrients that help the body clean up old cells, metabolize hormones, and detoxify. They may also help to protect the body against cancer.

Brussels Sprouts Salad with Walnuts and Manchego

Melissa got the inspiration for this unusual raw Brussels sprouts recipe from Franny's in Brooklyn, her favorite neighborhood restaurant. Andrew Feinberg, the chef, uses at least twice as much olive oil, walnuts, and cheese as this recipe. Our skinnier salad is still fantastic and, we think, one of the best in this whole book. If you're leery of raw Brussels sprouts, don't be here. Slicing them ultrathin and marinating them in lemon and oil tenderizes and flavors them.

Prep Time: 15 minutes   **Makes:** 6 servings

10	ounces Brussels sprouts (1 container), trimmed
	Juice of ½ lemon
	Coarse sea salt or kosher salt and freshly ground black pepper
3	tablespoons extra virgin olive oil or more, to taste
1	cup chopped toasted walnuts
3	ounces grated Manchego or young pecorino cheese (or even Gruyère) (about ¾ cup)

1. In a food processor, using the thinnest slicing disk, slice the Brussels sprouts (they will fall apart into shreds). Alternately, using a knife, slice the sprouts as thinly as possible. Put the sprouts in a bowl and toss with the lemon juice and a generous pinch of salt and pepper. Let rest for 5 minutes.

2. Add the olive oil and toss well. Add the walnuts and cheese and toss gently. Taste and adjust seasonings. You can serve this immediately, but it gets better after an hour or so and will last for up to 3 days in the fridge.

Brown bag it with: pineapple chunks

THE BIG HITS
Brussels sprouts have vitamin C, folate, and fiber. So while you might be put off by how they look, there's no denying their nutritional value. But if we're talking value and nutrition, it's the walnuts that are really remarkable. Full of omega-3 essential fatty acids, which reduce inflammation and help the heart, walnuts also have protein, fiber, folate, and arginine, an amino acid that helps arteries stay supple, reducing the risk of a heart attack. Walnuts are meaty and flavorful, so they are also quite filling.

Blender Gazpacho

Some summer days are so hot, muggy, and oppressive that even chewing can feel like work. In Spain one solution is to blend salad into a cool, refreshing puree that slides down the throat like a vegetable smoothie. Although tomatoes form the backbone of most gazpacho recipes, cucumbers, green pepper, and onions deepen the flavors here, while olive oil adds a touch of richness. Vinegar adds a jolt of acidity. You could serve this in a bowl with a spoon, in a glass, or cute espresso cups if you're making this for company. For an even chillier version, blend in an ice cube or two.

Prep Time: 10 minutes   **Makes:** 2 servings

- 1   pint cherry tomatoes
- ¼   cup chopped green bell pepper
- 2   tablespoons chopped red onion
- 2   tablespoons extra virgin olive oil
- 1   tablespoon chopped fresh flat-leaf parsley
- 1   tablespoon chopped fresh cilantro
- ½   teaspoon sherry vinegar, plus additional
- ½   teaspoon ground black pepper, plus additional
- ¼   teaspoon coarse sea salt or kosher salt, plus additional
- 1   cucumber, peeled, halved, seeded (½ roughly chopped, ½ diced)

1. In a blender combine tomatoes, green bell pepper, onion, olive oil, parsley, cilantro, vinegar, black pepper, salt, and the chopped cucumber, plus ¼ cup cold water, reserving the diced cucumber for serving. Blend until smooth. Taste and adjust the seasoning, if necessary.

2. Transfer the mixture to a bowl. Stir in the diced cucumber and transfer to the refrigerator to chill before serving.

Brown bag it with: an olive roll and apricots

LUNCH: BROWN BAG

THE BIG HITS

Tomatoes and onions supply the body with cancer-fighting anti-inflammatory antioxidants. Both have fiber and vitamin C—as do the cucumber and green pepper. Onions have sulfur compounds that are good for the heart and flavonoids that may protect against lung cancer and asthma. All in all, when you drink a cup of gazpacho, you're drinking a super soup of nutrients.

Bulgur Salad with Scallions, Parsley, Cucumber, and Tomatoes

The great thing about bulgur and couscous is that you don't need to cook them. A soak in boiling water is all they require to plump up and soften. You can use either for this bright, zesty salad. Couscous, which is essentially tiny beads of pasta, gives a slightly more mellow flavor than bulgur, which is finely cracked wheat. This salad holds up really well even at room temperature, making it perfect for picnics or to take to work if you don't have access to a fridge on the job.

Prep Time: 15 minutes, plus 30 minutes soaking   **Makes:** 4 to 6 servings

1	cup bulgur wheat (or use whole wheat or regular couscous prepared according to the package directions)
1½	teaspoons coarse sea salt or kosher salt
1	cucumber, peeled and trimmed
2	tablespoons freshly squeezed lemon juice
2	tablespoons extra virgin olive oil
2	cups chopped fresh flat-leaf parsley (about 2 bunches)
1	pint cherry tomatoes, quartered
4	scallions, white and green parts, thinly sliced
	Freshly ground black pepper

1. Place the bulgur in a large bowl and cover with 1½ cups boiling water. Add the salt and cover the bowl. Let sit until the bulgur has absorbed most of the liquid, about 30 minutes.

2. Slice the cucumber in half lengthwise. Scoop out the seeds with a spoon. Chop the cucumber into small cubes.

3. When the bulgur is ready, add the lemon juice and olive oil and toss to combine. Fold in the cucumber, parsley, tomatoes, and scallions. Season to taste with pepper.

Brown bag it with: dried figs or apricots

THE BIG HITS

Even if the name "bulgur" isn't so appetizing (it rhymes with vulgar), it is worth eating. Bulgur is a complex carbohydrate, which we all need. It serves up protein, niacin (a B vitamin), and insoluble fiber, which helps reduce the risk of diabetes and heart disease. It also has plant-based estrogen (aka a phytoestrogen) called lignans; they're fiber compounds that have antiviral, antibacterial, and antifungal properties.

Watermelon, Feta, and Olive Salad

The juxtaposition of cool, sweet watermelon and salty olives and feta makes a very satisfying lunch or snack. This salad won't last more than three or four hours after you toss it because the watermelon gets watery, which makes the whole thing soupy. So if you plan to take it to work for lunch, mix everything except the watermelon in one container and then add the melon just before you're ready to eat. If you can't find ripe watermelon, a combination of cucumber and cantaloupe makes an excellent substitution.

Prep Time: 10 minutes **Makes:** 1 serving

- 2 cups watermelon, cut into small chunks
- 1½ ounces feta cheese, crumbled (about ⅓ cup)
- 2 tablespoons chopped, pitted kalamata olives
- 2 tablespoons extra virgin olive oil
- 1 tablespoon chopped fresh herbs, such as basil or oregano, optional
  Coarse sea salt or kosher salt and freshly ground black pepper

1. Toss the watermelon, cheese, olives, oil, and, if desired, herbs together in a bowl. Season to taste with salt and pepper. Serve.

Brown bag it with: flatbread

THE BIG HITS

Watermelon is full of water, which means it's very filling. It's also delicious and full of vitamin C, beta-carotene, and B vitamins. Pink watermelon has the antioxidant lycopene, which is especially potent in fighting prostate cancer. The feta has calcium, of course, and the olives have those good monounsaturated fats.

Prosciutto, Mozzarella, Breadsticks, Cherry Tomatoes, and Celery Sticks

This instant, no-cook lunch is like an antipasti platter from your favorite Italian restaurant, except that you're probably going to be eating it in your kitchen. It tastes amazing no matter where you serve it.

Prep Time: 10 minutes **Makes:** 1 serving

- 2 ounces fresh mozzarella, cubed, or bocconcini balls (about ½ cup)
- 2 ounces thinly sliced prosciutto
  Extra virgin olive oil, for drizzling
  Coarse sea salt or kosher salt
- 1 cup cherry tomatoes
- 2 celery stalks, cut into sticks
  Bread sticks, for serving

1. In a small container combine the mozzarella and prosciutto. If your mozzarella is plain, you can give the mixture a drizzle of olive oil and a sprinkling of sea salt.

2. Place the cherry tomatoes and celery stalks in a separate container. Enjoy with breadsticks.

Brown bag it with: fresh fruit of your choice

THE BIG HITS

Between the tomatoes and the celery, this dish offers loads of vitamin C. The celery also has potassium, folate, and fiber, and the tomatoes have that antioxidizing lycopene. Mozzarella is a good source of protein, calcium, and selenium, which helps thyroid function and lowers the risk of joint inflammation.

Ultra-Garlicky Cumin Broccoli Salad with Tofu

With a ton of garlic, cumin, and chile flakes, this dish gives a huge flavor bang for the caloric buck. If you know dinner's going to happen on the couch with the TV on, make this ahead and try it instead of popcorn. It's zippier and better for you too. If you don't have cumin seeds on hand, leave them out.

Prep Time: 10 minutes, plus 1 hour marinating   **Makes:** 2 servings

- 1   head broccoli (about 1½ pounds), cut into bite-size florets (6 cups)
- ½   pound extrafirm tofu, cut into medium cubes (1½ cups)
- ½   teaspoon roasted (Asian) sesame oil
- 3   tablespoons extra virgin olive oil
- 3   garlic cloves, minced
- 1   teaspoon cumin seeds
- ½   teaspoon coarse sea salt or kosher salt, plus additional
      Pinch crushed red pepper flakes

1. Put the broccoli, tofu, and sesame oil in a large bowl and toss well.

2. In a large skillet heat the olive oil until hot but not smoking. Add the garlic and cumin and cook until fragrant, about 1 minute. Stir in the salt and pepper flakes. Pour the mixture over the broccoli and tofu and toss well. Let sit for at least 1 hour and up to 48 (pop it in the fridge if you want to keep it for more than 2 hours). Adjust seasonings (it may need more salt) and serve.

Brown bag it with: fresh fruit of your choice

THE BIG HITS

You'll be amazed by this dish's intense flavors, and it's so good for you, it's like going to the gym instead of shopping. What's so good? 1) Garlic has all these sulfur compounds that are good for your heart and help the body get rid of toxins. 2) Broccoli is full of antioxidants, potassium, and folate. Like garlic, it helps the body detoxify. It also has agents that kill ulcer-causing bacteria. 3) Soy is the best meatless protein around. It reduces cholesterol, helps maintain bones, and has choline, which improves memory. It's all good.

Roasted Cauliflower with Anchovies and Tapenade

Even if you know for sure you hate anchovies and cauliflower, try this recipe anyway. There is something about roasting the ingredients at high heat that works like alchemy, caramelizing and sweetening the cauliflower and transforming the anchovies into a happy, salty gilding that enhances all the other flavors without being the least bit assertive. It makes a great meatless entrée that's also quite filling. You could also substitute broccoli.

Prep Time: 35 minutes   **Makes:** 2 to 4 servings

- 1 head of cauliflower, trimmed, cored, and cut into bite-size pieces (about 4 cups)
- 1½ tablespoons extra virgin olive oil
  Coarse sea salt or kosher salt and freshly ground black pepper
- 2 anchovy fillets, finely chopped (about 1½ teaspoons)
- 1½ tablespoons olive tapenade or finely chopped kalamata olives
- 1 teaspoon freshly squeezed lemon juice
- 1 to 2 tablespoons chopped fresh parsley, optional

1. Preheat the oven to 400° F.

2. In a large bowl toss together the cauliflower and 1 tablespoon olive oil. Season to taste with salt and pepper and spread the cauliflower out in one layer on a baking sheet. Roast, tossing once or twice during cooking, until golden and tender, 25 to 30 minutes.

3. Meanwhile, in a small bowl whisk together the anchovies, tapenade, remaining ½ tablespoon olive oil, and the lemon juice.

4. Transfer the cauliflower to a bowl and add the anchovy mixture. Toss to combine and, if desired, garnish with chopped parsley. Serve warm or at room temperature.

Brown bag it with: a ciabatta roll and pineapple

THE BIG HITS

Olives are always a good choice because of their monounsaturated fats, and studies have shown that people who eat diets rich in olives and olive oil have a lower risk of heart disease. Cauliflower has a lot of vitamin C and a fair amount of the B vitamin folate. It also keeps for a really long time in your fridge, so it's a good fallback veggie when you can only get to the market once a week.

Boiled Greens Salad with Olives, Lemon, and Feta

Use whatever greens you want for this recipe. We think Swiss chard is the easiest to clean because you can just slice off all the stems in one fell swoop, whereas you have to pull each stem individually from kale, collard, and mustard green leaves, which takes a few minutes. Then again, these heartier, thicker greens have a punchier flavor than chard.

Prep Time: 20 minutes   **Makes:** 2 servings

- 1 large bunch kale, Swiss chard, collard, mustard, or other greens ($3/4$ pound), thick stems discarded, torn into pieces
- $1\frac{1}{2}$ tablespoons freshly squeezed lemon juice
  Pinch crushed red pepper flakes
- $\frac{1}{2}$ teaspoon coarse sea salt or kosher salt, plus additional
- 2 tablespoons extra virgin olive oil
- 2 to 3 ounces feta cheese, cut into cubes (about $\frac{1}{2}$ to $\frac{3}{4}$ cup)
- $\frac{1}{2}$ cup grape tomatoes, halved, optional
- $\frac{1}{4}$ cup kalamata olives, pitted and sliced
  Whole wheat pita, toasted, for serving

1. Bring a large pot of salted water to a boil and add the greens. Cook until just tender, 2 to 6 minutes, depending on the type of green (the tougher the green, the longer the cooking time), then drain well, pressing out the excess liquid.

2. In a large bowl whisk together the lemon juice, red pepper flakes, and salt. Whisk in the oil. Add the greens, toss well, then top with the feta, tomatoes, and olives. Serve with whole wheat pita.

Brown bag it with: a whole wheat pita and fresh fruit

THE BIG HITS

It's the leafy greens that pack the biggest nutritional punch in this recipe. They're full of fiber, calcium, and folate, which may help fight heart disease and certain cancers. Everyone knows calcium is good for your bones, but did you know calcium helps the heart maintain a regular rhythm and helps nerve impulses to transmit properly? Women ages 19 to 50 need 1,000 mg a day, and women over 50 need 1,200 mg a day. It's not easy to get that much calcium, but these greens will help.

Snacks & Sweets

Somewhat-Lighter Baba Ganouj with Yogurt

We like this light, flavorful dip even better than non-*Skinny* baba ganouj recipes. It has a much fluffier texture that still sticks to cut-up veggies and a pleasant kick, thanks to the cayenne. Plus, we can eat more of it and still save room for cookies.

Prep Time: 10 minutes, plus 25 minutes cooking   **Makes:** 4 to 6 servings

- 1   medium eggplant, trimmed, peeled, and cubed
- 2   tablespoons extra virgin olive oil
- 1   teaspoon coarse sea salt or kosher salt, plus additional
- ¼   teaspoon cayenne pepper
- ½   cup low-fat Greek yogurt
- 1   tablespoon tahini
- 1   tablespoon freshly squeezed lemon juice
- 1   scallion, white and green parts, trimmed and thinly sliced
- 1   garlic clove, minced
-     Pita chips, for serving

1. Preheat the oven to 400°F. In a medium bowl toss the eggplant with the olive oil, salt, and cayenne.

2. Spread out the eggplant in an even layer on a large baking sheet. Roast, tossing occasionally, until tender and golden, about 25 minutes. Let cool for 5 minutes.

3. In a food processor combine the roasted eggplant and yogurt, tahini, lemon juice, scallion, and garlic and blend until smooth. Taste and adjust the seasonings, if necessary. Serve with pita chips.

SNACKS & SWEETS

THE BIG HITS

There's no baba ganouj without eggplant, so here's a look at the nutritional contributions it makes to your body. First, it's loaded with dietary fiber. Since we require 25 to 30 grams of fiber per day, and most Americans only get 14 to 15 grams, you're in luck with this dip. Eggplant also has a number of powerful antioxidants. One, nasunin, seems to protect the fats (lipids) in brain cell membranes. And both the yogurt and tahini (ground sesame seeds) in this baba give a girl some always-needed calcium.

Half-and-Half Guacamole

Upping the tomato content of guacamole turns an occasional treat into an everyday snack—especially if you're serving it with carrot sticks.

Prep Time: 15 minutes **Makes:** 2 servings

- 1 ripe avocado, pitted and peeled
- ½ cup chopped tomato
- 2 tablespoons prepared salsa, plus additional, to taste
- ¼ teaspoon coarse sea salt or kosher salt and freshly ground black pepper
  Lime juice, optional
  Carrot sticks and tortilla chips, for serving

1. Slice the avocado in half lengthwise. Placing the avocado halves on a flat surface, plunge the tip of a sharp knife into the pit. Turn the knife clockwise, dislodging the pit. Use a spoon to scoop out the avocado flesh into a medium bowl; mash it well with a fork. Fold in the tomato, salsa, salt, and pepper.

2. Taste the guacamole and adjust the seasonings, adding lime juice, if necessary. Serve immediately with carrot sticks.

THE BIG HITS

Avocados are a natural source of monounsaturated fat, which is the fat that lowers bad (LDL) cholesterol levels. It not only has carotenoids (antioxidants that are potentially protective against breast cancer), it has other substances that help the body absorb them better. Ounce for ounce, an avocado has 60 percent more potassium than the famous-for-its-potassium banana. Plus it has fiber, folate, vitamin E, and iron. And all the tomatoes here will give you even more fiber, vitamin C, and the antioxidant lycopene.

Addictive Spiced Popcorn

Piquant and crunchy, this won't bore you even if you eat it all. Luckily you can eat a lot of popcorn without guilt. Leftovers, if there are any, will keep for a week when stored airtight at room temperature. A resealable plastic freezer bag works well.

Prep Time: 10 minutes **Makes:** 4 servings

- 1½ tablespoons extra virgin olive oil
- 1 teaspoon sweet paprika
- ¼ teaspoon coarse sea salt or kosher salt
- ⅛ teaspoon ground cumin
- Tiny pinch cayenne
- ½ cup popcorn kernels

1. In a large pot over medium-high heat combine oil, paprika, salt, cumin, cayenne, and popcorn. Stir well, coating the popcorn kernels evenly with the oil and spices.

2. Cover the pot and shake back and forth over the burner until most of the kernels have popped (the popping should slow to one pop every 2 seconds), 3 to 5 minutes.

3. Transfer the popcorn immediately to a serving bowl. Taste; adjust the seasoning, if necessary.

SNACKS & SWEETS

THE BIG HITS

Sure, there's a lot of fiber in popcorn. But let's be honest: The real value of popcorn is that you can eat a lot of it and not worry about the calories. And sometimes, no matter how aware you are, how interested in the joy of eating you are, you just want to sit down with a big, honking bowl of popcorn.

Chile Pumpkin Seeds

Not only are these incredibly tasty, they're actually good for you. They're perfect to have on hand when a salt craving strikes and your body really needs something more nutritious than, say, potato chips.

Prep Time: 5 minutes   **Makes:** ³⁄₄ cup

- 1 tablespoon extra virgin olive oil
- ³⁄₄ cup hulled pumpkin seeds
- ³⁄₄ teaspoon ground cumin
- Pinch cayenne pepper
- Fine sea salt or kosher salt

1. To make the pumpkin seeds, in a small skillet over medium high heat, heat the oil. Add the pumpkin seeds and cook until the seeds begin to pop, 1 to 2 minutes.

2. Add the cumin and cayenne and continue to cook until fragrant, about 30 seconds more. Season with a generous pinch of salt.

THE BIG HITS

Pumpkin seeds may be small, but they pack a big nutritional punch. Granted, one of the biggest benefits seems to be in reducing the risk of prostate cancer, but they also are rich in zinc, which helps bones stay dense, and have protein, iron, and antioxidants. In some parts of the world, they're thought of as an aphrodisiac. What could be bad about adding this little extra zing? The rewards could be so, ahem, satisfying.

Crispy Sesame Tofu Sticks

Salty, crispy, and spicy, these tofu sticks will satisfy that BBQ potato chip craving in a more nutritious manner. Leftovers are terrific on top of a spinach salad. Almost like bacon. Almost.

Prep Time: 20 minutes **Makes:** 2 to 4 servings

- 1 (14-ounce) package extrafirm tofu, drained
- ⅓ cup soy sauce
- 2 teaspoons roasted (Asian) sesame oil
- 1 teaspoon chile oil or Tabasco
- 2 tablespoons chopped scallions, white and light green parts only, optional

1. Preheat the broiler.

2. Slice the tofu crosswise into ½-inch slabs, then halve the slabs into sticks. To drain, place the tofu on a baking sheet lined with a double layer of paper towels. Cover the tofu with another double layer of paper towels and place another, slightly smaller, baking sheet on top. Place a heavy can on top of the tray to weight it down.

3. In a small bowl whisk together the soy sauce, sesame oil, and chile oil.

4. Remove the can, the smaller baking sheet, and all the paper towels from the large baking sheet. Using a pastry brush or a spoon, cover the tofu generously with half of the soy mixture. Transfer the tofu to the oven and broil until slightly dry to the touch, 8 to 10 minutes. Add the scallions to the remaining sauce, if desired, and serve the tofu with the sauce for dipping.

SNACKS & SWEETS

THE BIG HITS
Soy has fiber, omega-3 essential fatty acids, potassium, and choline, which helps the liver clean the body of toxins, stops the buildup of cholesterol, and produces memory-enhancing chemicals. Soy, like meat, is a complete protein. But unlike meat, it's low in saturated fat. Some people think that eating too much soy can cause hormonal imbalances, thyroid problems, and allergies. So here's the thing: Eat it in moderation. If you like it, eat reasonably sized servings of it. Don't eat soy at every meal. For that matter, don't eat any one food at every meal.

Roasted Peaches with Black Pepper, Brown Sugar, and Balsamic

This makes a perfect snack for when you don't know what will satisfy that Need-Something-Now! pang somewhere between lunch and dinner (or breakfast and lunch, for that matter). If you want to make them a full-fledged dessert, up the sugar to 3 tablespoons and serve them over frozen yogurt. You can substitute nectarines if those are riper than the peaches.

Prep Time: 10 minutes, plus 25 minutes roasting   **Makes:** 2 servings

- 1 tablespoon unsalted butter, softened
- 2 tablespoons dark brown sugar
  Coarse sea salt or kosher salt and freshly ground black pepper
- 4 ripe peaches, halved and pitted
- 2 teaspoons balsamic vinegar
  Vanilla frozen yogurt or ice cream, for serving, optional

1. Preheat oven to 375°F. In a small bowl mash together the butter, sugar, and a pinch each of salt and pepper.

2. Spoon the mixture into the cavities of the peach halves and arrange the peaches on a rimmed baking pan, stuffed sides up. Spoon ¼ teaspoon balsamic over each peach half. Bake until the peaches are softened and the butter is bubbling, about 25 minutes. Serve hot, warm, or at room temperature with yogurt or ice cream, if desired.

SNACKS & SWEETS

THE BIG HITS

Peaches. They have fiber (eat the peel), antioxidizing vitamin C, and vitamin A, which aids the body in making white blood cells, helps maintain regular cell growth and division, and helps keep your bones healthy. Peaches also serve up calcium—about 6 milligrams in a medium fruit.

Roasted Pears with Chestnut Honey

Roasting the pears in chestnut honey gives this dish a nice robust flavor, but if you don't have any around or don't feel like seeking it out at a specialty store, regular honey works well too. The sprinkling of cinnamon on top is a classic with the pears, but feel free to flavor this dish any way you'd like—our variation using black pepper and thyme lends the pears an unexpected sweet and savory twist.

Be sure to use firm Bosc pears here. Other varieties tend to fall apart.

Prep Time: 15 minutes   **Makes:** 2 servings

- 2   tablespoons chestnut or other full-flavored honey, such as buckwheat, or regular honey
- 2   firm Bosc pears, quartered and cored
- 2   teaspoons unsalted butter
   Pinch ground cinnamon, optional
   Freshly ground black pepper, optional
   Sprig fresh thyme, optional

SNACKS & SWEETS

1. Preheat the oven to 350°F.

2. In an oven-safe pan large enough to hold the pears in a single layer simmer the honey over medium-high heat until slightly thickened, about 2 minutes.

3. Place the pears, cut sides up, and the butter in the pan. Sprinkle with the cinnamon, if desired. Reduce the heat to low and cover the pan. Cook, turning and basting once or twice, until pale golden and not quite tender, 5 to 7 minutes.

4. Transfer the pan to the oven and continue to roast, turning once or twice, until golden brown and tender, 5 to 7 minutes more. Serve warm or at room temperature, drizzled with the honey from the pan. If desired, season with black pepper and fresh thyme.

THE BIG HITS

Pears are full of vitamin C, copper (an antioxidant), and fiber. Even though it seems like most fruits and vegetables have a good amount of fiber, the truth is most of us just don't eat enough of it, so eat more whenever you can. Fiber lowers cholesterol and helps the body digest food more slowly, which keeps you feeling full longer. Besides, for a dessert or snack that's "good for you," these honey-roasted pears feel like a great big treat.

Dinner

Watercress or Arugula Salad with Avocado, Goat Cheese, and Lime

Not only are salads made with dark leafy greens like watercress and arugula better for you than, say, iceberg lettuce, they have a tart, spicy taste that holds its own when combined with the lime juice and goat cheese. We added some avocado to smooth out and tame the flavors in this recipe. It's a good go-to salad when you know your body needs something healthful but you crave something decadent.

Prep Time: 15 minutes   **Makes:** 1 to 2 servings

- 1 tablespoon extra virgin olive oil
- 2 teaspoons freshly squeezed lime juice
- 1 bunch watercress (about 4 cups) or 2 bunches arugula
- ½ avocado, cubed
- 1½ ounces goat cheese, crumbled (about ⅓ cup)
- Coarse sea salt or kosher salt and freshly ground black pepper

1. Whisk together the olive oil and lime juice in a small bowl.

2. Toss together the watercress and the lime vinaigrette in a medium bowl. Add the avocado and goat cheese and toss gently to combine. Season to taste with salt and pepper.

DINNER

THE BIG HITS

If you make this salad with arugula, you're choosing a dark leafy green that happens to be a cruciferous vegetable like broccoli or cauliflower. As a cruciferous vegetable, arugula has the phytochemicals known as indoles, which may help prevent cancer. They also have calcium, folate, some beta-carotene, and more vitamin C than any other salad green. All in all, a good choice.

Caesar Salad to Die (But Not Get Fat) For

We love Caesar salad, but when we order it, we often get a gloppy, bland dish that's not worth the calories. Here is our antidote to all the awful Caesars out there. It's pungent from anchovies, Parmesan, and garlic, crisp from croutons and romaine lettuce hearts, and creamy from the egg yolk. The extra dressing can be stored in an airtight container in the refrigerator for up to 5 days.

Prep Time: 25 minutes **Makes:** 2 to 4 servings

For the Salad:

- 1 cup whole wheat or white bread cubes (stale bread works best)
- 1 tablespoon extra virgin olive oil
  Coarse sea salt or kosher salt
- 2 eggs
- 1 head romaine lettuce, outer leaves discarded, torn into pieces
- 2 ounces grated Parmesan cheese (about ¼ cup)

For the Dressing:

- 4 to 6 anchovy fillets (or more, to taste)
  Freshly squeezed juice of ½ lemon
- 1 garlic clove, passed through a garlic press or minced
- ⅛ teaspoon Worcestershire sauce
- 2 dashes Tabasco
  Coarse sea salt or kosher salt and freshly ground black pepper
- ¼ cup extra virgin olive oil

1. To make the salad, preheat the oven to 300°F. Toss the bread cubes with the oil and season with the salt. Spread the bread in a single layer on a baking sheet and toast until golden brown, 12 to 15 minutes. Let cool.

2. Bring a small pot of water to a boil. Add the eggs and cook for 1½ minutes. Drain and let cool.

3. To make the dressing, place the first six ingredients in a blender and blend to combine. With the blender running, slowly add the olive oil until fully incorporated. Taste. Adjust the seasoning, if necessary.

4. Place the salad greens in a large bowl. Crack the eggs and add to the bowl, breaking the eggs up slightly with a fork. Add the croutons, cheese, and just enough dressing to coat the greens lightly.

DINNER

THE BIG HITS

Studies have shown that when you enjoy your food, you process the nutrients more efficiently so you get more of the good stuff out of what you eat. So what nutrients are in this extremely enjoyable salad? From the dressing, you get raw garlic, which is full of sulfur compounds that are good for your cardiovascular health. The greens have folate and other B vitamins, fiber, vitamin C (an antioxidant), and beta-carotene (also an antioxidant).

Curly Chicory Salad with Bacon and Egg

Curly chicory isn't the kind of green you'll usually find made into salad. Its slight bitterness can be a turnoff to the timid. But adding rich ingredients, such as crispy bacon and soft-cooked eggs, softens and mellows its intensity, and its ruffled leaves are ideal for trapping all drips of runny yolk. It's a terrific, filling main-dish salad.

Prep Time: 15 minutes   **Makes:** 2 servings

- 2 eggs
- 3 slices bacon
- 1 bunch curly chicory, long stems removed, leafy greens torn into bite-size pieces (about 8 cups greens)
- 1 tablespoon extra virgin olive oil
- 1½ teaspoons freshly squeezed lemon juice, or to taste
  Coarse sea salt or kosher salt and freshly ground black pepper

1. Bring a small saucepan of water to a boil. Add the eggs and cook for 4 minutes. Drain and let the eggs cool.

2. In a medium pan over medium-high heat cook the bacon until crisp. With a slotted spoon transfer the bacon to a plate lined with paper towels. Reserve ½ tablespoon of the fat from the pan. When the bacon is cool enough to handle, cut it into ½-inch pieces.

3. Wash the greens well and spin dry in a salad spinner. Place them in a large bowl. Add the reserved bacon fat, oil, and lemon juice and toss to combine. Peel the cooled eggs and add to the salad, breaking up lightly with a fork. Season the salad with salt and pepper, to taste, toss again, and serve.

DINNER

THE BIG HITS

Curly chicory, like its more familiar cousins radicchio and endive (the sleek, rocket-shape kind), is rich in iron and vitamins A, C, and K, which helps blood clot and bones form and repair, among other things. An egg is packed with protein and choline, which is good for your brain cells and nerves. And bacon, well, if you eat it and crave it, bacon is simply good for your soul. In sum, this dish is a little decadent and a lot good for you.

Roasted Eggplant, Peppers, Onions, and Cherry Tomatoes with an Egg on Top

This is our cheater's version of ratatouille. Instead of sauteing the vegetables in lots of olive oil for a long time, here we toss them with just enough oil to slick them down, then roast them at high heat. Not only is it quicker and easier, it's less oily and much fresher tasting too. And we love the crunchy, olive-oil-fried egg on top.

Prep Time: 20 minutes, plus 25 to 30 minutes roasting

Makes: 2 to 4 servings

1	large eggplant (about 1¼ pounds), trimmed and cubed
1	pint cherry tomatoes
2	small red bell peppers, cored and cubed
2	small red onions, cubed
3	tablespoons extra virgin olive oil
1	teaspoon coarse sea salt or kosher salt, plus additional
½	teaspoon ground black pepper, plus additional
2	tablespoons finely chopped fresh basil
2	to 4 eggs

1. Preheat the oven to 400°F. In a large bowl toss together the eggplant, tomatoes, bell peppers, onions, 2 tablespoons olive oil, salt, and pepper.

2. Spread the vegetables in a single layer on a baking sheet. Roast until tender and golden brown, 25 to 30 minutes. Toss with the basil.

3. To make the eggs, in a skillet large enough to fit all of the eggs (or working in batches, if necessary) heat the remaining tablespoon oil. Crack the eggs into the skillet and cook until the bottoms are crispy and brown but the yolks are runny. Season with salt and pepper.

4. Divide the roasted vegetables among individual serving plates and top each plate with a fried egg.

DINNER

THE BIG HITS

Eggplants have a huge amount of fiber as well as phytonutrients (plant-based nutrients) that keep your cell membranes healthy and your cholesterol levels low. Red onions are especially full of heart-healthy sulfur compounds, as well as folate and calcium. If you choose to add an egg, you'll be adding a complete protein that's relatively low in saturated fat. Plus eggs are an excellent source of a nutrient called choline, which the body needs for brain and nerve functions.

Sauteed Green Beans with Bacon, Black Pepper, and Cherry Tomatoes

Filled with chunks of bacon and juicy cherry tomatoes, this savory green bean dish easily makes a light meal on its own, maybe served with some crusty bread or roasted potatoes. If you want to gild the lily, try frying up some eggs in olive oil (see page 194) and sliding them on top.

Prep Time: 25 minutes **Makes:** 2 to 4 servings

- 3 slices bacon, diced (about 1/4 cup)
- 1 small red onion, thinly sliced
- 1 pound green beans, trimmed (about 4 cups)
- 1 pint cherry tomatoes, halved (about 1 1/2 cups)
  Coarse sea salt or kosher salt and freshly ground black pepper

1. In a large skillet cook and stir the bacon over medium-high heat until most of the fat has rendered, about 4 minutes. Add the onion and cook, stirring, until the onion is well browned, 5 to 7 minutes.

2. Add 2 tablespoons water to the pan, let cook for 1 minute, then add the green beans and cherry tomatoes. Reduce the heat to low, cover the pan, and cook, stirring occasionally, until the beans are tender, 8 to 10 minutes.

3. Season the beans with salt and a generous amount of pepper and serve.

DINNER

THE BIG HITS

You might be wondering what bacon is doing in a book that's all about keeping your body happy and little-black-dress-ready over the long haul. Truth be told, unless you're a vegetarian or keep kosher or halal, there's no reason to not eat some bacon every now and again. Like all intensely flavored high-fat foods, a little goes a long way—and a little bacon never hurt anyone. Besides, this dish is still full of good stuff like lycopene and vitamin C in the cherry tomatoes and fiber, vitamin K, and vitamin C in the green beans.

Sesame-Roasted Mushrooms with Soba

Served either hot or at room temperature, this dish is great mounded on top of hearty greens like arugula, watercress, or baby spinach.

Prep Time: 30 minutes   **Makes:** 6 servings

- 1   pound shiitake or cremini mushrooms, stems removed, caps thinly sliced (about 6 cups)
- 2   tablespoons extra virgin olive oil
- 2   tablespoons roasted (Asian) sesame oil
  Coarse sea salt or kosher salt and freshly ground black pepper
- 1   (12-ounce) package buckwheat soba noodles
- 3   tablespoons Japanese shoyu or soy sauce
- 1   bunch scallions, white and light green parts thinly sliced (about ³/₄ cup)
- ½   cup chopped fresh cilantro
  Sesame seeds, toasted, optional, for garnish
  Lime or lemon wedges, for serving

1. Preheat the oven to 400°F.

2. Spread the mushrooms out on a baking sheet and toss with the olive oil and 1 tablespoon of the sesame oil. Season with a large pinch of salt and pepper. Roast in the oven until the mushrooms are slightly crisp and golden, about 20 minutes.

3. Bring a large pot of water to a boil. Add the soba noodles and cook until just al dente, checking occasionally to see that they do not overcook, about 6 minutes. Transfer to a colander to drain and immediately rinse with cold water. Let drain completely.

4. Toss the noodles with the shoyu or soy sauce and the remaining 1 tablespoon of sesame oil in a bowl. Add the scallions and cilantro and toss to combine.

5. Transfer the noodles to a platter or individual serving plates and top with the mushrooms. Sprinkle with sesame seeds and, if desired, serve with lime wedges.

DINNER

THE BIG HITS

Shiitake mushrooms are the most widely cultivated mushroom in the world. They have a substance called lentinan in them. It both invigorates your immune system and potentially lowers your risk of cancer. Soba noodles are made from buckwheat. A serving of soba (which is a little less than a cup) has 5 grams of protein—that's about how much protein is in an egg. Soba also has fiber and various B vitamins, especially folate.

Roasted Tofu with Shiitake, Soy, and Ginger over Baby Spinach

Roasted marinated tofu is one of those addictive foods that's OK to keep eating, compared to say, cheese fondue or doughnut holes. The combination of shiitake mushrooms and soy makes our version particularly hearty.

Prep Time: 20 minutes, plus 40 minutes cooking **Makes:** 2 to 4 servings

- 6 tablespoons soy sauce
- 6 tablespoons rice wine vinegar
- 3 tablespoons extra virgin olive oil
- 2½ tablespoons honey
- 2½ tablespoons minced gingerroot
- 2 cloves garlic, minced
- ¾ pound shiitake mushrooms, wiped clean and stems removed (you can substitute sliced button mushrooms)
- 1 pound firm tofu, rinsed, patted dry, and sliced ½ inch thick
- 1 quart baby spinach leaves

1. Preheat the oven to 375°F.

2. In a bowl whisk together the soy sauce, vinegar, oil, honey, ginger, and garlic. Place the mushrooms in a bowl and add enough of the marinade to evenly coat them. Toss to combine.

3. Arrange the tofu in a single layer in a small baking dish. Pour the remaining marinade over the tofu.

4. Transfer the tofu to the oven and roast for 20 minutes. Spread the mushrooms out on one or two baking sheets and transfer to the oven. Continue roasting the tofu and the mushrooms until the tofu is nearly dry and well browned and the mushrooms are tender and golden, about 10 to 15 minutes.

5. Arrange the spinach on serving plates. Drizzle with some of the remaining marinade from the tofu pan. Divide the tofu slices among the plates and top with some of the mushrooms. Serve.

DINNER

THE BIG HITS

Soy is the only plant-based complete protein and, unlike meat, it doesn't have saturated fat. It does have a lot of nutrients—omega-3 essential fatty acids, calcium, fiber, choline, folate, and more. Shiitake mushrooms are full of antioxidants and a variety of substances that boost your immune system, lower your cholesterol, and potentially lower your risk of cancer. Spinach has folate, fiber, beta-carotene, and calcium, among other nutrients.

Hot Cinnamon-Glazed Sweet Potatoes with Yogurt

Soft baked sweet potatoes, glazed with cinnamon and a pinch of cayenne and topped with plain yogurt, are filing enough for a meatless meal. We love these served with the Pan-Seared Brussels Sprouts on page 166.

Prep Time: 30 minutes   Makes: 2 to 4 servings

- 1½   tablespoons unsalted butter (or use olive oil)
- ¾   teaspoon ground cinnamon
-   Pinch cayenne
- 2   medium sweet potatoes, scrubbed and cut into medium cubes
-   Coarse sea salt or kosher salt and freshly ground black pepper
-   Plain yogurt, for serving

1. Preheat the oven to 400°F. In a large saucepan over medium heat melt the butter. Remove from the heat and stir in the cinnamon and cayenne. (Or just mix the olive oil and spices in a large bowl.)

2. Add the potatoes to the spice mixture and toss to combine; season with salt and pepper to taste and toss again. Spread the potatoes out in an even layer on a rimmed baking sheet.

3. Transfer the potatoes to the oven and roast, stirring once or twice during cooking, until fork tender, 20 to 25 minutes. Serve the potatoes hot with a dollop of yogurt on top.

DINNER

THE BIG HITS

Sweet potatoes couldn't be better for you. Rich with the anitoxidant beta-carotene, they also have vitamin C, folate, magnesium (which assists in—count 'em—300 functions in the body), and potassium (along with other stuff). They rate fairly low on the Glycemic Index, which means that the amount of carbs in any one serving of sweet potato is relatively low, especially when compared with white potatoes. And did we mention they taste so good?

Quick Kale and White Bean Soup

Somewhere between a soup and a stew, this hearty, comforting dish is made for rainy, chilly evenings. Serve it with thick slices of toasted country bread lightly slicked with extra virgin olive oil and feel free to dunk!

Prep Time: 20 minutes   **Makes:** 4 servings

- 1   bunch kale, stems removed
- 1½   tablespoons extra virgin olive oil, plus additional, for serving, optional
- 1   onion, finely chopped
- 2   garlic cloves, minced
- 3   (15.5 ounce) cans cannellini beans, rinsed and drained
- 1   quart chicken stock or broth
- ¾   teaspoon coarse sea salt or kosher salt
  Pinch red pepper flakes
  Freshly ground black pepper
  Olive oil, optional
  Finely grated Parmesan cheese, for serving, optional

1. Lay some of the kale leaves one on top of the other to make a small stack. Roll them up into a cigar and slice crosswise into strips. Repeat with remaining kale.

2. In a large pot heat 1½ tablespoons olive oil over medium-high heat. Add the onion and garlic and saute until softened, about 5 minutes. Add the beans, kale, chicken stock, salt, red pepper flakes, and black pepper to taste. Simmer, stirring occasionally, until the kale is cooked through, about 15 minutes.

3. Using a potato masher or wooden spoon, mash the beans slightly in the pot and serve. For a richer flavor, continue to simmer until the soup thickens and becomes more stewlike. Divide into serving bowls and top with a drizzle of olive oil and a sprinkle of grated cheese, if using.

DINNER

THE BIG HITS

Kale: It's leafy and it's green. This means it has folate, beta-carotene, and, like spinach, lots of calcium. It also has potassium and a huge serving of vitamin A. It apparently also has some cancer-fighting sulfur compounds. So don't limit your interaction with kale to home decoration, though the plants do look lovely in window boxes.

Curried Vegetable Lentil Soup

Loaded with vegetables and served with lime wedges, this lentil soup is lighter, more colorful, and all-around perkier than most. But it's still perfect for a cold winter Sunday meal.

Prep Time: 20 minutes, plus 30 minutes to 1 hour cooking

Makes: 4 servings

- 1½ tablespoons extra virgin olive oil
- 1 onion, halved and thinly sliced crosswise
- 1 to 2 tablespoons curry powder, to taste
- 2 medium carrots, diced small (about ½ cup)
- ½ red bell pepper, diced small (about ⅔ cup)
- 1 medium zucchini, diced medium (about 1¼ cups)
- 1 cup lentils, rinsed under cold running water and drained
- 1 quart chicken stock or broth
- ½ cup finely chopped fresh cilantro
  Coarse sea salt or kosher salt and freshly ground black pepper
  Lime wedges, for serving

1. Heat the oil in a large pot over medium heat. Add the onion and curry powder and cook, stirring, until the onion begins to brown, 7 to 10 minutes. Add the carrots, bell pepper, and zucchini and continue to cook and stir until the vegetables begin to soften, about 5 minutes more. If at any time the curry or onion starts to look too brown (that is, dark brown in places), reduce the heat.

2. Add the lentils and chicken stock and bring the mixture to a boil. Reduce the heat to a simmer and cook, stirring occasionally, until the lentils are tender and the soup has thickened, 30 minutes to 1 hour, depending on the age of the lentils. Older lentils take longer to cook.

3. Stir in the cilantro and add salt and black pepper to taste. Ladle into bowls and serve with lime wedges.

DINNER

THE BIG HITS

Lentils are a legume like chickpeas, peas, and beans. Like those foods, lentils are a good source of protein and fiber. In fact when it comes to fiber, the little lentil leads the pack. Specifically, it's full of soluble fiber, which when mixed with water, forms a gel-like substance and takes bad (LDL) cholesterol right out of you.

Spicy Chickpea and Tomato Stew with Spinach

This is one of those dishes that's completely adaptable to season and circumstance. If it's summer and you have some nice ripe tomatoes on your counter, use them. If it's winter, use canned tomatoes. Ditto the spinach. Use a bag of fresh baby spinach or choose frozen spinach. And if you don't have canned chickpeas, use whichever beans you have on hand.

Prep Time: 20 minutes   **Makes:** 2 servings

- 2 tablespoons extra virgin olive oil
- ¼ teaspoon hot paprika (or use sweet paprika and a pinch of cayenne)
- 2 garlic cloves, minced
- 1 large red onion, sliced
- ½ teaspoon ground coriander
  Coarse sea salt or kosher salt and freshly ground black pepper
- 1 can (15 ounces) chickpeas, drained
- 2 large tomatoes, cored and diced, or 1 pint cherry or grape tomatoes, diced, or 1 can (15 ounces) diced tomatoes
- 4 cups baby spinach or 1 package (10 ounces) frozen spinach
  Sherry or white wine vinegar, to taste

1. In a pot heat the oil over high heat. Add the paprika and cook for 30 seconds. Add the garlic and let cook until it turns opaque and smells garlicky, about 30 seconds. Add the onion, coriander, and a generous pinch of salt and pepper; cook and stir until the onion softens, about 5 minutes.

2. Stir in the chickpeas and tomatoes, partially cover the pot, and let the mixture simmer until the tomatoes thicken up slightly, about 10 minutes. Add water, a tablespoon at a time, if the mixture seems too dry. Stir in the spinach and cook until it wilts or defrosts. Season with vinegar, to taste, and serve hot.

DINNER

THE BIG HITS

It's all good in this vegetarian stew. Cooking tomatoes makes the nutrient lycopene, an antioxidant, easier for the body to process. Chickpeas are a legume with protein, folate, and fiber, all of which just might protect you against heart disease and cancer. And the spinach? It has (among other good things) iron, zinc, vitamin C, and folate. You name it, spinach has it—and so does this dish.

Roasted Salmon with Carrots, Molasses, and Chile

This recipe works equally well with parsnips, turnips, or rutabaga. If you have fresh herbs in your fridge, chop them up and use them as a garnish. Tarragon, basil, cilantro, and parsley would be our first choices, though rosemary and thyme are nice too. If you want to add something green and crunchy, try slicing up an endive and serving it alongside. It's a nice cool counterpart to the spicy carrots and requires little effort since the endive is easy to rinse, dry, and slice.

Prep Time: 15 minutes, plus 25 to 30 minutes roasting   **Makes:** 2 servings

1	pound carrots (usually 1 bunch without the greens)
2	tablespoons extra virgin olive oil
2	tablespoons molasses
	Pinch cayenne
	Sea salt or kosher salt and freshly ground black pepper
2	salmon fillets, 4 to 6 ounces each
	Chopped fresh herbs, optional, for garnish
	Lemon wedges, for serving

1. Preheat the oven to 375°F. Peel the carrots and slice them on a bias (this is prettier than coins and no more work) about ¾ inch thick.

2. In a large bowl whisk together 1½ tablespoons of the oil, the molasses, cayenne, and a generous pinch of salt and pepper. Add the carrot slices and toss well. Spread the mixture out on a rimmed baking sheet and roast, stirring once or twice, until golden and tender, 25 to 30 minutes.

3. Season the salmon with salt and pepper and rub with the remaining ½ tablespoon of olive oil. Place the fish on a small baking pan and pop it in the oven with the carrots during the last 10 minutes. The fish is done when it's opaque on the top but still darker pink inside, 8 to 10 minutes depending upon how thick the fillets are. You should be able to cut into it with a fork, but it shouldn't flake (that's overdone).

4. Serve the salmon and carrots garnished with herbs, if you have them, and lemon wedges.

DINNER

THE BIG HITS

Salmon is rich in omega-3 essential fatty acids, which reduce inflammation in the body. There's debate about the dangers of salmon, particularly from PCBs, which can be found in both wild and farmed fish. Eat salmon at most once a week and buy the best you can (avoid farmed Atlantic salmon). Carrots have vitamin A, which helps your vision. And molasses is full of iron, which helps prevent anemia.

Seared Tuna or Halibut with Parsley and Dried Tomato Salad

Parsley leaves make a very intense, full-flavored salad that's a little like watercress but without the bitterness. Along with the pungent dried tomatoes, it's a great match for meaty seared fish steaks, such as tuna or halibut, or even salmon. Leftovers are wonderful stuffed into a pita.

Prep Time: 20 minutes **Makes:** 2 servings

- 1 tablespoon extra virgin olive oil
- 1 teaspoon soy sauce
- 2 (4- to 6-ounce) tuna or halibut steaks, about 1 inch thick
  Coarse sea salt or kosher salt and freshly ground black pepper
- 1 large bunch flat-leaf parsley, rinsed
- 2 tablespoons very thinly sliced oil-packed dried tomatoes
- 1 teaspoon freshly squeezed lemon juice

1. In a small bowl whisk together the olive oil and soy sauce. Rub the mixture into the tuna steaks. Season the tuna with salt and pepper.

2. Heat a medium pan over medium heat until very hot. Place the tuna steaks in the pan and sear (without moving) until golden brown, about 3 to 5 minutes per side, to taste.

3. To make the salad, twist the stems from the parsley. In a bowl toss together the parsley, tomatoes, and lemon juice. Season with salt and pepper to taste. Divide the salad between two serving plates and place a tuna steak on top of each salad. Serve.

DINNER

THE BIG HITS

Fish can carry pollutants—specifically, methylmercury and PCBs (in farmed salmon)—from the waters they swim in and the foods they eat. But fish is an excellent source of lean protein. As consumers, what do we do? Avoid fish with high mercury levels (swordfish, shark, king mackerel, tilefish). Eat a variety of fish and only eat about 12 ounces a week. Buy the best you can afford. (We like wild Pacific salmon, if you can find it.) For help on what fish to buy, see "The Fish List" on page 144.

Roasted Halibut or Hake with Zucchini and Mint Pesto

The mint pesto in this yummy roasted fish dish is too small a batch for the food processor, but if you'd like to use one, double or triple the recipe. The extra pesto will keep in an airtight container in the refrigerator for up to 2 weeks. Once you have it around, you'll want to use it on everything: vegetables, meats, chicken, other seafood, eggs, or even in sandwiches. Try substituting basil for the mint, which makes the recipe more traditionally pestolike, albeit still without the cheese and nuts.

Prep Time: 20 minutes, plus 20 to 25 minutes roasting **Makes:** 2 servings

- 3 tablespoons fresh mint leaves, chopped
- 2 garlic cloves, peeled
- 3 teaspoons extra virgin olive oil, plus extra for brushing
- ¼ teaspoon coarse sea salt or kosher salt, plus additional
- 2 small zucchini, trimmed and cut lengthwise into ¼-inch slices
   Freshly ground black pepper
- 2 (8-ounce) halibut or hake fillets
   Plain yogurt or lemon wedges, for serving

1. Preheat oven to 450°F. To make the pesto, use a mortar and pestle to pound together the mint, 1 garlic clove, 1 teaspoon of the oil, and ¼ teaspoon salt until it forms a paste. (If you do not have a mortar and pestle, use a sharp large knife to finely chop the mint, garlic, and salt until you almost have paste, then combine it in a bowl with the oil.)

2. Arrange the zucchini in a single layer on a baking sheet and lightly brush with some more of the olive oil. Season with salt and pepper. Roast until the zucchini is golden brown around the edges, 20 to 25 minutes.

3. Meanwhile, prepare the fish. Place the fillets on a baking sheet, rub each fillet with the garlic clove, then drizzle with the remaining 2 teaspoons of olive oil and season with salt and pepper. Transfer the fish to the oven along with the zucchini and roast until just cooked through and flaking, 7 to 10 minutes, depending on the thickness of the fish.

4. To serve, toss the zucchini with the pesto and arrange on two serving plates. Place one fish fillet on top of each plate. Garnish with a dollop of plain yogurt or a lemon wedge, if desired.

DINNER

THE BIG HITS

We'll be honest, zucchini has a lot of water, and it's not the most nutritious vegetable in the garden patch. But it does OK. It has vitamin C, fiber, folate, magnesium, and vitamin A and is an excellent part of a heart-smart eating plan. Mint, just sprinkled here, has been used throughout history to soothe digestive ills. And fish is always a good choice for protein because it's so lean.

Pan-Seared Red Snapper with Chunky Cherry Tomato Sauce and Garlic

If you can get cherry tomatoes in an assortment of colors (red, yellow, and orange), this ridiculously easy after-work snapper dish morphs into something fancy enough for company. If you want to substitute a higher-rent fish such as black sea bass fillets for the snapper while you're at it, go right ahead.

Prep Time: 20 minutes **Makes:** 2 servings

- 2 (6-ounce) skinless red snapper fillets, rinsed and patted dry
  Coarse sea salt or kosher salt and freshly ground black pepper
- 2 tablespoons extra virgin olive oil
- 2 garlic cloves, minced
- 1 pint cherry tomatoes, halved
- 1½ tablespoons chopped fresh sage

1. Season both sides of the fish with salt and pepper.

2. In a large pan over medium-high heat warm 1 tablespoon of the oil. Add the garlic and cook, stirring, until golden, about 1 minute. Add the tomatoes and sage and continue to cook until the tomatoes have softened and form a chunky sauce, 7 to 10 minutes. Adjust the heat, if necessary, to prevent burning. Spoon the tomato mixture into a bowl and cover to keep warm.

3. Add the remaining tablespoon oil to the pan and heat until hot but not smoking. Place the fish fillets in the pan and cook, without moving, until the bottom is golden brown, about 3 minutes. Turn the fish and cook the other side until the fillet is opaque, 1 to 2 minutes more.

4. Transfer the fish to two serving plates and spoon the tomatoes on top of the fish. Serve hot.

DINNER

THE BIG HITS

Tomatoes have vitamin C, sure, but they also have lycopene, a carotenoid that has potentially cancer-fighting properties and may help fight heart disease. When tomatoes are cooked, they lose water, which intensifies the lycopene, making it easier for the body to process. Garlic is famously good for you—all those sulfur compounds will keep the heart healthy. And any high- or low-rent fish is an excellent source of lean protein.

Seared Garlicky Squid or Shrimp over Mixed Greens

If you've never made squid, this is the perfect initiation recipe because sauteing these quick-cooking cephalopods with garlic is about the easiest thing in the world. Your squid will come already cleaned. You can ask your fishmonger to make sure if there's any doubt. All you have to do is slice each squid in thirds crosswise before tossing them in the saute pan. Or substitute shrimp, which are a more familiar but more expensive choice.

Prep Time: 15 minutes   **Makes:** 2 servings

- ½   pound cleaned squid or large shrimp, peeled and deveined
- 2   tablespoons extra virgin olive oil
- 2   garlic cloves, minced
- Pinch of crushed red pepper flakes
- Coarse sea salt or kosher salt
- 1   quart mixed greens, for serving
- Freshly squeezed lemon juice

1. If using squid, slice each one crosswise into thirds. If using shrimp, halve each one crosswise. In a pan large enough to hold the squid or shrimp in a single layer heat the olive oil over medium-high heat. Add the garlic and pepper flakes and cook, stirring, for 30 seconds.

2. Add the squid or shrimp to the pan and season with a large pinch of salt. Cook, stirring, until just opaque, about 2 minutes (do not overcook).

3. Arrange the salad greens on a platter or individual serving plates. Top with the cooked squid or shrimp and the oil from the pan. Drizzle lemon juice over all and sprinkle with more salt and/or pepper flakes to taste. Serve hot.

DINNER

THE BIG HITS

Garlicky anything is good for you. Studies suggest that people who eat a lot of garlic have lower rates of heart disease and stomach cancer. It's the sulfur compounds in garlic that provide these benefits. The antioxidant selenium and a substance called allicin don't hurt, either. When you cook garlic, you lose some of its health benefits, but others remain because certain of its sulfur compounds are converted into different, still beneficial compounds.

Roasted Chicken Thighs with Sherried Grapes and Watercress

If you've never had roasted grapes, you're in for a huge treat. The high heat of the oven caramelizes their skins and condenses their juices, giving you a sweet-tart, soft-yet-raisinlike fruit that's just amazing seasoned with a little sherry vinegar and served with roasted chicken. Make this once and we guarantee you'll make it again. If you want to get fancy, use a mix of grapes: black, red, and green—just make sure they're all seedless. If not, at least don't forget to warn your guests!

Prep Time: 10 minutes, plus 20 to 25 minutes roasting   **Makes:** 2 servings

- 4 chicken thighs (about 1½ pounds)
- 1 garlic clove, halved
- 1½ tablespoons extra virgin olive oil
  Coarse sea salt or kosher salt and freshly ground black pepper
- 1 pound seedless red grapes
- 3 tablespoons sherry vinegar
- 1 tablespoon unsalted butter (or use olive oil)
- ½ teaspoon sugar
- 1 bunch watercress, stems removed

1. Preheat the oven to 450°F.

2. Rub each chicken piece all over with the garlic clove. Toss the chicken with 1 tablespoon of the olive oil and season with a large pinch of salt and pepper. Transfer the chicken to one side of a large rimmed baking sheet.

3. In a medium bowl toss together the grapes, vinegar, butter, and sugar. Season the mixture with a large pinch of salt and pepper. Spread the grapes out on the other half of the baking sheet.

4. Roast the chicken and the grapes, tossing the grapes occasionally, until the chicken skin is crispy and the juices run clear when pierced with a fork, 20 to 25 minutes.

5. Toss the watercress with the remaining ½ tablespoon olive oil. Arrange the watercress on a platter or individual serving plates and place the chicken on top. Spoon the grapes over the chicken and serve.

DINNER

THE BIG HITS

Fresh or roasted, grapes have a heart-protecting flavonoid (a chemical compound found in plants) called quercetin; vitamin C; and the mineral manganese, which helps the enzymes in the body. Watercress is chockfull of vitamins C, B_1, K, and E, plus iron, calcium, zinc, and beta-carotene; and, like those grapes, it also has the flavonoid quercetin. Fill up your plate with watercress; it's so good for your body.

Roasted Chicken Breasts with Rosemary Apples

Melissa got the inspiration for this dish while she was working on a cookbook with David Bouley, who serves a more complicated apple-rosemary sauce as one of the many garnishes on a dish of oil-poached salmon. Streamlined and paired with roasted chicken breasts, it's easy enough for a midweek dinner but is still interesting and delectable enough to serve to company. You could also stay truer to Bouley's vision and substitute salmon for the chicken, reducing the cooking time to 7 to 10 minutes because fish cooks faster than fowl.

Prep Time: 25 minutes   **Makes:** 2 servings

- 2 boneless, skinless chicken breasts (about 6 to 7 ounces each)
- ½ garlic clove
- ½ tablespoon extra virgin olive oil
  Coarse sea salt or kosher salt and freshly ground black pepper
- 1 tablespoon unsalted butter (or use olive oil)
- 2 large Granny Smith apples, peeled, cored, and coarsely chopped (about 2½ cups)
- 2 tablespoons white wine or water
- 1 large sprig rosemary

1. Preheat the oven to 400°F. Rub each chicken breast with garlic. Drizzle with the olive oil and season with salt and pepper. Transfer to a rimmed baking sheet and roast until the juices run clear, about 20 minutes.

2. Meanwhile, make the apples: In a medium saucepan over medium-high heat melt the butter. Cook until golden brown, 1 to 2 minutes.

3. Add the apples, wine or water, and rosemary. Reduce the heat to medium-low, cover, and cook, shaking the pan occasionally, until the apples are tender and have broken down slightly, about 15 minutes. (If the pan juices dry out before the apples are soft, add another tablespoon or two of water and keep cooking.) Remove the rosemary sprig and season the sauce with salt and a generous amount of pepper.

4. Arrange the chicken on individual serving plates and spoon the apples on top. Serve hot.

THE BIG HITS

Here's a little refresher on why chicken is a good choice in a healthy diet. A 4-ounce serving gives you about 67 percent of your daily protein requirement, and the fat is less saturated than the fat in red meat. Of course, when you eat the skin (which you don't in this recipe), you double the amount of fat—so only eat the skin when it's absolutely irresistibly prepared (e.g., crisp and golden).

DINNER

Turkey or Pork Sausage with Spicy Sauteed Broccoli Rabe

If you aren't in the mood for sausages, leave them out and skip step two. If you take the sausage-free route, you might want to add an extra garlic clove or more crushed red pepper and then finish the dish with a downpour of cheese instead of the usual sprinkle; otherwise you might miss the meat. If you don't want to use wine, water is perfectly fine. If you do use wine, a dry white wine is tart and puckery, vermouth makes it slightly herbaceous, and dry sherry tastes a bit nutty. If you only have cream sherry, that's fine too. The sweetness is actually nice with the bitter greens.

Prep Time: 20 minutes **Makes:** 2 to 4 servings

- 2 bunches broccoli rabe (about 1 pound each)
- 1 pound sausages of your choice, sliced 1 inch thick
- 1 tablespoon extra virgin olive oil
- 2 garlic cloves, minced
  Pinch of crushed red pepper flakes
- ¼ cup white wine, vermouth, sherry, or water
  Coarse sea salt or kosher salt and freshly ground black pepper
  Grated Parmesan or pecorino cheese

1. Rinse the rabe and, using a paring knife, trim most of the leaves and the thick stem from each stalk. You can keep the tender part of the stem; just get rid of the tough bottoms.

2. Heat a large skillet over medium heat, then toss in the sausage slices. Cook, stirring once or twice, until browned, about 5 minutes.

3. When the sausage is brown all over, add the oil, garlic, and pepper flakes. Saute for a few seconds until the garlic turns opaque and smells garlicky. Add broccoli rabe and wine or water, bring to a simmer while stirring, then cover the pan. Let simmer for 3 minutes, then uncover and cook until all the liquid evaporates, about 2 minutes longer. Season with salt, black pepper, and cheese. Serve immediately.

DINNER

THE BIG HITS

Broccoli rabe has beta-carotene; the antioxidant, immune-system-boosting vitamin C; and a big serving of fiber. This dish also serves up garlic, which studies have shown can help lower LDL (bad) cholesterol levels. Garlic also has antioxidants that are potentially cancer-fighting.

London Broil with Caramelized Pineapple

If you have time, marinate the steak in the garlic paste. Rub the steak all over with the paste, wrap it in plastic, and refrigerate it for as much time as you have —anywhere from 30 minutes up to 24 hours.

Prep Time: 30 minutes   **Makes:** 6 servings

- 1   large pineapple, trimmed, peeled, and cored
- 1   tablespoon plus 2 teaspoons extra virgin olive oil
- 1   teaspoon sugar
  Tabasco sauce, to taste
- 1   garlic clove
- ½   teaspoon coarse sea salt or kosher salt, plus additional
- ½   teaspoon ground black pepper
- 1   (2-pound) London broil, skirt, or flank steak (about 1 to 1½ inches thick)
- 1   head radicchio, halved, cored, and thinly sliced crosswise into shreds
  Chopped fresh parsley, basil, or cilantro, for garnish (optional)

1. Preheat the oven to broil. Slice the pineapple into quarters lengthwise. Cut the quarters crosswise into large bite-size pieces, about ½-inch chunks.

2. In a bowl combine the pineapple, 2 teaspoons olive oil, sugar, and Tabasco sauce. Spread the pineapple out on a baking sheet. Transfer it to the oven and broil until the pineapple is caramelized and golden brown, 7 to 10 minutes.

3. Meanwhile, run the garlic clove through a garlic press or chop it as finely as possible. Mix with the remaining 1 tablespoon olive oil, ½ teaspoon salt, and the pepper to form a paste. Rub the paste all over the steak and place the steak on a baking sheet.

4. When the pineapple is cooked, transfer it to a bowl. Add the sliced radicchio, season to taste with salt, and toss well.

5. Transfer the steak to the oven and broil, turning once, 3 to 6 minutes per side or until desired doneness. Remove from the oven and let rest 10 minutes before slicing very thinly crosswise against the grain.

6. Arrange the radicchio and pineapple on a platter or individual serving plates. Top with slices of meat and, if desired, garnish with the herbs.

DINNER

THE BIG HITS

As you'd expect from the tart, tangy, tropical pineapple, it has a lot of vitamin C and fiber. It also has manganese, which works with antioxidants to rein in all those free radicals. Radicchio offers potassium and magnesium as well as vitamin A. The unexpected combination of the two offers you plenty of pleasure.

Instant Recipes
Frozen/Prepared

Instant Coleslaw

The hardest part of making coleslaw is shredding the cabbage and carrots. Luckily the folks who revolutionized our lives with prewashed salad in a bag did the same thing for coleslaw, making it extremely quick to whip up. Our version is a bit lighter than usual (of course) and much tangier from the generous dollops of Dijon mustard and lemon juice.

Prep Time: 5 minutes   **Makes:** 2 servings

- ½   of 1 (16-ounce) bag shredded cabbage mix
- 1   tablespoon mayonnaise
- 1   tablespoon extra virgin olive oil
- 2   teaspoons Dijon mustard
- 2   teaspoons freshly squeezed lemon juice
- 1   large pinch celery or caraway seeds, optional
  Pinch coarse sea salt or kosher salt
  Freshly ground black pepper

1. Place the cabbage mix in a bowl.

2. In a separate bowl whisk together the mayonnaise, olive oil, mustard, and lemon juice. Pour over the cabbage mixture and toss to combine. Add the celery seeds, if using, and season the slaw with salt and pepper, to taste. Serve.

THE BIG HITS

Cabbage is cheap and widely available, which is good because it happens to be really good for you. It has vitamin C and both soluble and insoluble fiber. It's a cruciferous vegetable, and like other such veggies (broccoli, cauliflower, Brussels sprouts), it has micronutrients known as indoles, which may lower the risk of some kinds of cancer.

Fast Winter Squash Soup with Lime

Although this soup takes about a half hour to simmer into a luxurious puree, putting it together is about as fast as you can get. It makes an incredibly easy and tasty starter for a Thanksgiving meal. If you really want to jazz it up, serve it topped with some of the Chile Pumpkin Seeds on page 186.

Prep Time: 40 minutes   Makes: 4 servings

- 1   tablespoon unsalted butter or olive oil
- 1   medium red onion, finely chopped
- 2   (12-ounce) packages frozen cooked winter squash
- 3   cups low-sodium chicken broth
     Finely grated zest of one lime
     Freshly squeezed juice of half a lime
- ½   teaspoon coarse sea salt or kosher salt
- ½   teaspoon freshly ground black pepper
     Chile Pumpkin Seeds (page 186), optional

1. In a medium saucepan over medium-high heat melt the butter or heat the oil. Saute the onion until translucent, about 3 minutes. Add the squash and the broth and bring to a boil.

2. Reduce the heat and simmer until the soup thickens, 30 to 35 minutes. Add the lime zest and juice and season with salt and pepper.

3. Ladle the soup into bowls, garnish with the pumpkin seeds, if desired, and serve.

INSTANT RECIPES

THE BIG HITS

Winter squashes are full of vitamin A, a compound that dissolves in fat and helps your vision, skin, bone growth, and cell division; vitamin C; potassium, which helps keep your fluids balanced; and fiber. Orange winter squashes have the antioxidant beta-carotene—the deeper the orange color, the more of the nutrient.

Edamame with Sesame and Soy Sauce

If you've only sucked the beans out of edamame pods in Japanese restaurants, this recipe is something else entirely. Quickly cooked frozen beans stay crisp and just need a little bit of soy, sesame oil, and rice wine vinegar to bring out the flavor. They make a hearty snack or instant lunch and can even be dinner if you serve them over brown or white rice. Just keep the portion of carbs small, meaning under a cup. If you like, add some cubed tofu. If you don't have soy, vinegar, and sesame oil, just cook the beans in a little chicken broth or a rehydrated bouillon cube.

Prep Time: 10 minutes   **Makes:** 2 servings

> 2   teaspoons soy sauce
> 2   teaspoons rice wine or white wine vinegar
> 1½   teaspoons roasted (Asian) sesame oil
> 2   cups frozen shelled edamame
>   Sliced scallions, for garnish, optional
>   Coarse sea salt or kosher salt, optional

1. In a pot whisk together the soy sauce, rice wine vinegar, and sesame oil. Add the edamame and bring to a simmer. Cover the pot.

2. Once the edamame are tender, 1 to 5 minutes depending on the brand, turn off the heat. Garnish with the scallions and salt, if desired.

INSTANT RECIPES

THE BIG HITS
Say it: Soy, Soy, Soy! Edamame are soybeans, which means they have protein, fiber, choline (good for your brain and nerves), calcium, selenium (which mixes with proteins and becomes an antioxidizing agent), and folate. Soy fights cancer and heart disease and is ridiculously good for you.

Seared Artichoke Hearts with Pecorino and Basil

Frozen artichoke hearts are an absolute boon for the time-pressed cook. They're cleaned and precooked; all you have to do is defrost and saute, in this case with a little fresh basil and some pecorino or Parmesan cheese. We love this for lunch with some crusty bread drizzled with olive oil and salt or for dinner over some whole wheat pasta—but not too much, about 1 cup cooked. It's also a terrific side dish for chicken or fish.

Prep Time: 10 minutes   **Makes:** 1 to 2 servings

- 1 **tablespoon extra virgin olive oil**
  Pinch crushed red pepper flakes
- 1 **(9-ounce) package frozen artichoke hearts, defrosted**
- 1 **ounce grated pecorino or Parmesan cheese (about ¼ cup)**
  Coarse sea salt or kosher salt and freshly ground black pepper
- 2 **tablespoons chopped fresh basil**
  Lemon wedges, for serving

1. In a pan large enough to hold the artichokes in a single layer heat the olive oil over medium-high heat until hot but not smoking. Add the red pepper flakes and cook until fragrant, about 30 seconds.

2. Add the artichokes, cut sides down, and sear, without moving, until the bottoms are brown, about 5 minutes. Flip the artichokes and brown the other sides, about 2 minutes more.

3. Sprinkle the artichokes with the cheese and cook until the cheese has melted and begins to turn golden, about 3 minutes. Season the artichokes with salt and pepper and transfer to a bowl. Toss with the basil. Transfer to serving plates and serve with lemon wedges.

INSTANT RECIPES

THE BIG HITS

The artichoke has fiber, folate, vitamin C, many minerals, and even some protein. It's true that many people steer clear of this veggie because the fresh ones can be so hard to negotiate. But with the frozen hearts, there's no reason not to partake, and the health benefits are ample.

Okra, Cherry Tomato, and Corn Saute

Frozen okra is one of those convenience foods that is arguably even better than fresh. Because the packagers precook it before freezing, they rid the pods of much of their mucilaginous texture, which a lot of people don't like. Here we mixed okra with frozen corn and fresh tomatoes for a summery saute that's in season all year long. Serve it as a side dish for grilled meat or fish or as a main dish when your body needs an all-veggie meal.

Prep Time: 15 minutes   **Makes:** 2 to 4 servings

1 tablespoon extra virgin olive oil
1 small yellow onion, sliced
½ teaspoon coarse sea salt or kosher salt
1 pint cherry tomatoes, halved
1 (10-ounce) package frozen okra
1 cup frozen corn
  Freshly ground black pepper
1 teaspoon freshly squeezed lime juice
1 tablespoon chopped fresh cilantro
1 tablespoon chopped fresh flat-leaf parsley

1. In a large saute pan over high heat, heat the olive oil. Add the onion and salt and cook and stir until golden brown, about 5 minutes (adjust the heat, if necessary, so that the onion doesn't burn).

2. Stir in the tomatoes, okra, and corn and cook, stirring, until the vegetables are heated through, 7 to 10 minutes. Season with pepper and stir in the lime juice, cilantro, and parsley. Serve.

INSTANT RECIPES

THE BIG HITS

Okra is widely eaten throughout the world. From a nutritional point of view, there are good reasons for its popularity. It has vitamin C, folate, and other B vitamins, as well as potassium. It also has magnesium, which the body needs for more than 300 biochemical reactions. Among other functions, it helps keep heart rhythm steady, supports a healthy immune system, helps regulate blood sugar levels, and keeps bones strong.

Sauteed Broccoli with Red Pepper Flakes

When Melissa hits the top of her 2-pound limit for weight gain, she makes this recipe. It's filling enough for dinner, yet it's heartier and more satisfying than a salad. Of course, if you would rather use fresh broccoli, go right ahead. Blanch it first by giving it a 1-minute dip in boiling water or microwave it until it turns bright green, then proceed with the recipe. If you are craving a little protein with this, round it out with cubed tofu or cooked chicken.

Prep Time: 5 minutes **Makes:** 1 serving

- 1 tablespoon extra virgin olive oil
- 1 garlic clove, minced
   Pinch crushed red pepper flakes
- 1 (10-ounce) package frozen broccoli, defrosted
   Coarse sea salt or kosher salt

1. Heat the olive oil in a medium skillet over medium-high heat. Add the garlic and pepper flakes and cook until the garlic begins to turn golden and smells garlicky, about 30 seconds.

2. Add the broccoli and salt, to taste, and cook, stirring, until the broccoli is heated through, 2 to 3 minutes.

INSTANT RECIPES

THE BIG HITS

You might think it's nuts to make a meal of just broccoli, but from a nutritional standpoint, it's a great choice. Broccoli is full of folate, which helps you produce and maintain new cells; vitamin C for immune boosting and antioxidizing; vitamin A, which improves vision and skin; and vitamin K, good for your blood and heart. It also contains fiber and a range of cancer-fighting phytonutrients.

Sugar Snap Peas with Mint

If it's sugar snap season, substitute fresh for the frozen. Just give them a quick dip in boiling water (about 1 minute), then drain and proceed with the recipe.

Prep Time: 5 minutes   **Makes:** 2 to 4 servings

- 1 (8-ounce) package sugar snap peas, defrosted and drained
- 1 teaspoon extra virgin olive oil
- ½ teaspoon freshly squeezed lemon juice
- 1 tablespoon chopped fresh mint
- **Coarse sea salt or kosher salt and freshly ground black pepper**

1. Toss the peas, olive oil, and lemon juice in a bowl. Add the mint and toss again to combine. Season with salt and pepper. Serve chilled or at room temperature.

THE BIG HITS

Sugar snap peas are an edible pod. They have iron, potassium, some B vitamins (thiamin, niacin, riboflavin), vitamin C, potassium, and vitamin A. What do these nutrients do? Iron helps red blood cell production; potassium and thiamin aid in the normal functioning of nerves (among other things); vitamin C is an antioxidant and may bolster your immune system; and vitamin A helps keep the lining of your eyes and respiratory, urinary, and intestinal tracts healthy.

Sauteed Green Beans with Pecans

This is about as tasty as frozen vegetables can get.

Prep Time: 5 minutes **Makes:** 2 to 4 servings

- 1 tablespoon unsalted butter or extra virgin olive oil
- 2 tablespoons chopped pecans, toasted
- 1 garlic clove, finely chopped
- 1 (9-ounce) package frozen French-cut green beans, defrosted and drained

  Coarse sea salt or kosher salt and freshly ground black pepper

1. In a medium skillet over medium-high heat melt the butter. Add the pecans and garlic and cook and stir until both are golden and fragrant, 2 to 3 minutes.

2. Stir in the green beans and cook until heated through. Season with salt and pepper.

INSTANT RECIPES

THE BIG HITS

Green beans are full of fiber, vitamin C, and vitamin K, which helps the body absorb calcium (among other things). They serve up other nutrients like folate, potassium, magnesium, and even some calcium. Pecans, like most nuts, are extremely nutritious. They have a lot of protein, iron, potassium, and fiber. They also contain B vitamins thiamin, niacin, and riboflavin. Of course, nuts also have a fair amount of fat, so be a little moderate with them.

Garlicky Spinach and Yogurt Dip with Dill

When we tested this recipe, which is supposed to feed four as a snack, the two of us devoured the whole bowl—on virtuous rye crisp crackers at least—in about 6 minutes flat. Can you say lunch? With a supercreamy texture from the Greek yogurt, plus a nice jolt of garlic and dill, it's even better than the mayonnaise-drenched spinach dips we adore (in much greater moderation). If you're having a party, make a triple batch at least. It's that good!

Prep Time: 10 minutes **Makes:** 4 servings

- 1 (10-ounce) package frozen chopped spinach, defrosted and drained
- 1 cup Greek yogurt
- 1 small garlic clove, minced
- 1 tablespoon chopped fresh dill
- Coarse sea salt or kosher salt and freshly ground black pepper
- Crudités, crackers, or pita chips, for serving

1. Combine the spinach, yogurt, garlic, and dill in a bowl. Season to taste with salt and pepper. Serve with crudités, crackers, or pita chips.

INSTANT RECIPES

THE BIG HITS

There's a reason spinach made Popeye strong. Spinach has iron, potassium, folate, beta-carotene (that dark color), vitamins C and K, fiber, and various micronutrients. But the good stuff in this dip doesn't end with the spinach. The garlic has sulfur compounds that are excellent for your heart. And then there's the calcium- and protein-rich yogurt. No matter how much of this dip you eat, you get something good from every bite.

Instant Recipes – Takeout

Steamed Mixed Vegetables with Asian Dipping Sauce

Most of the time when you order steamed mixed vegetables from your standby Chinese take-out joint, they just give you soy sauce for dipping. This version is a slightly more exciting alternative. It's also great for dipping cubes of raw tofu, if you have a block tucked away in the fridge.

Prep Time: 5 minutes   **Makes:** 1 to 2 servings

- 1 order steamed mixed vegetables from your favorite restaurant
- 1 tablespoon soy sauce
- 1 tablespoon rice wine vinegar
- 1 tablespoon roasted (Asian) sesame oil

1. In a small bowl whisk together the soy sauce, vinegar, and sesame oil. Transfer the vegetables to a plate and serve with the bowl of dipping sauce.

INSTANT RECIPES

THE BIG HITS

The value of this dish is obvious: You don't have to cook. You can order in Chinese food and eat a meal that isn't drenched in oil and grease. And whatever vegetables you get will have loads of fiber and vitamins.

Steamed Mixed Vegetables with Blue Cheese

Although blue cheese is assertive, its salty flavor makes it stellar with mixed veggies. Goat cheese or grated Parmesan makes a tasty substitute.

Prep Time: 5 minutes   **Makes:** 1 to 2 servings

- 1   order steamed mixed vegetables from your favorite restaurant
- 2   ounces blue cheese, crumbled (about ½ cup)

1. Place your veggies in a bowl and toss with the cheese. Eat hot or at room temperature.

INSTANT RECIPES

THE BIG HITS

Of course you get calcium and protein from the cheese, no matter what kind you choose. You also know that you'll have a satisfying dinner—and the only prep time is mostly the wait for the delivery guy.

Pad Thai and Baby Spinach Salad

Who doesn't love a big bowl of soft, silky pad thai noodles topped with peanuts, bits of egg, and shrimp? But who can justify eating an entire order without possibly doing damage to her little black dress figure? Here's a win-win situation: Bulk the pad Thai out with baby spinach and cucumber and only eat a quarter of it. The sauce flavors the vegetables and lightens the noodles, and the cucumbers (or daikon radish) add an appealing crunch. Another great thing about this dish is that it works just as well if your pad Thai arrives hot or has cooled down. Hot pad Thai wilts the spinach and cooks it slightly, while cold pad Thai keeps it more saladlike. Both ways are delicious. This is also an ideally healthful way to stretch leftovers.

Prep Time: 10 minutes   **Makes:** 4 to 6 servings

- 1 order pad Thai from your favorite take-out place (or substitute lo mein)
- 2 (5-ounce) bags baby spinach
- 1 cup thinly sliced cucumber or daikon radish

1. In a large bowl toss together the pad Thai, spinach, and cucumber. Enjoy hot or at room temperature.

THE BIG HITS

This is a brilliant way to eat more spinach, and because spinach is so incredibly good for you, there's no reason not to eat as much of it as you possibly can. It has iron, calcium, folate, fiber, and many vitamins. In fact, if you're over 30 and eat spinach every day, its folate might help reduce your risk of stroke.

Cold Sesame Noodles and Cucumber Salad

This is similar to the pad Thai recipe on page 224 but even richer, thanks to the sesame paste in the sauce. It holds up well for a buffet if you're serving a crowd; just multiply the recipe as necessary.

Prep Time: 5 minutes   **Makes:** 4 servings

- 1 order sesame soba noodles from your favorite Oriental take-out place
- 1 English cucumber, trimmed, halved, and thinly sliced into half moons
- 2 scallions, white and green parts, trimmed and thinly sliced

1. In a bowl toss together the noodles and cucumber. Divide the mixture among individual serving plates and top with sliced scallions.

THE BIG HITS

A photo of a woman lying back with her hair wrapped in a towel, a white skin-care mask on her face, and cucumbers over her eyes is, of course, a spa cliche. But the stuff in cucumbers (silica, caffeic acid, ascorbic acid—aka vitamin C) that soothes skin from the outside is also good for skin and connective tissue on the inside. Plus, there's a lot of fiber and water in cucumbers, and we all need more of both.

Seared Sashimi à la Nobu

We got the idea for this from Nobu restaurant, where one of chef Nobu Matsuhisa's signature recipes involves searing his sashimi for a few seconds. It's a terrific variation on the same old sashimi from your local sushi joint, and is also a perfect way to use any leftover sashimi or sushi in the fridge. Serve it with a side of oshitashi (boiled spinach or watercress) or a nice big salad to make sure you get your veggies in.

Prep Time: 5 minutes   Makes: 1 to 2 servings

- 1 tablespoon soy sauce
- 1 tablespoon freshly squeezed lemon juice
- 1 tablespoon extra virgin olive oil
- 1 order sashimi from your favorite Japanese take-out place

1. In a small bowl stir together the soy sauce and lemon juice.

2. Heat the olive oil in a medium pan over high heat until very hot but not smoking. Place the sashimi pieces in the pan and sear them on one side, without moving, until crisp and golden, about 30 seconds. Do not cook them all the way through.

3. Transfer the fish to a plate. Serve the sashimi with the soy and lemon mixture for dipping.

INSTANT RECIPES

THE BIG HITS

Whichever kind of fish you have in your jeweled array of sashimi, each slice will have something good for you. Full of vitamins and minerals, fish is an excellent source of complete protein and, unlike red meat, is low in heart-clogging saturated fat. Fish also has omega-3 essential fatty acids, which studies have shown are good for your heart.

The Skinny 2-Week Meal Plan

Jump-start your life on The Skinny

We know we keep telling you to start living *The Skinny* life the very next time you're hungry. But we also know that changing your eating lifestyle is harder than just saying, "OK, I'm always going to have salad for lunch." (We know. We've tried.)

So to help you slip into new habits (and favorite little black dresses) more comfortably, we've outlined two weeks' worth of meals. There's no science behind these daily menus—eating these exact meals won't do anything to your cells other than give them many delicious nutrients to digest.

Use the meal plan as a guide to help you figure out how you can adapt your tastes, habits, and needs to life on *The Skinny*. Don't worry, we have you covered no matter what your cooking style. If you're in the mood to cook at home, check out the "make it" options. If all you have time for is takeout, check out the "don't make it" options.

WEEK ONE

Day 1

BREAKFAST:

Make It: Ginger-Stewed Rhubarb with Yogurt (page 151). Serve yourself 1 cup; sprinkle on a teaspoon or two of chopped nuts if you need some crunch.

Don't Make It: Substitute fresh fruit for the rhubarb.

LUNCH:

Make It: Ultra Garlicky Cumin Broccoli Salad with Tofu (page 179) and an apple or other fruit

Don't Make It: Lightly dressed vegetable salad with some type of protein (4 to 6 ounces, or a fist-size portion, of chicken, fish, nuts, cheese, whatever) and an apple or other fruit

DINNER:

Make It: Roasted Salmon with Carrots, Molasses, and Chile (page 202), with ½ cup Israeli or whole wheat couscous

Sort of Make It: Roasted salmon (follow instructions on page 202), a salad, and a small whole grain roll or whole wheat tortilla or flatbread

Don't Make It: Order in some sashimi and Japanese vegetables (ask for brown rice).

DESSERT:

You pick (keep an eye on those portions!) or have some fruit.

SNACKS (midmorning or midafternoon; always optional):

Tea, banana, Somewhat-Lighter Baba Ganouj with Yogurt (page 183) and a few baked pita chips, or a small piece of cheese with celery sticks

Day 2

BREAKFAST:

Make It: Almond Butter and Strawberry Breakfast Smoothie (page 152), 1 cup

Don't Make It: 1 cup of whole grain cereal with fat-free soymilk, or rice milk and half a banana, sliced

LUNCH:

Make It: Tuna and Cucumber Salad with Olives (page 170), a whole grain roll, and a pear or other fruit

Don't Make It: Italian tuna salad (no mayo) from the gourmet shop or roasted/grilled salmon from a salad bar with greens and a whole grain roll

Don't Make It: Leftover salmon or Ultra-Garlicky Cumin Broccoli Salad with Tofu (page 179) with fruit

DINNER:

Make It: Roasted Chicken Thighs with Sherried Grapes and Watercress (page 207)

Don't Make It: Order in a lean (not fried) chicken and vegetable dish. (Any Middle Eastern places around?)

DESSERT:

Leftover Ginger-Stewed Rhubarb (page 151) with a dollop of yogurt, or a cookie (1 or 2, depending on the size)

SNACKS (midmorning or midafternoon; always optional):
Watermelon (sprinkle with mint if you're feeling fancy or salt if you're feeling feisty); a slice of whole grain toast with some butter; tea; or whatever you're craving

WEEK 1

Day 3

BREAKFAST:
Oatmeal (1 cup) topped with fresh fruit (or more leftover Ginger-Stewed Rhubarb) and a little (¼ cup) warm milk, if you'd like

LUNCH:
Make It: Chicken Salad (you can use leftover thighs if you have them) with Roasted Red Peppers (page 171) on whole wheat bread, grapes

Don't Make It: Turkey sandwich (hold the mayo, slap on the mustard) on whole wheat bread, grapes

DINNER:
Make It: Spicy Chickpea and Tomato Stew with Spinach (page 201)

Don't Make It: Store-bought vegetable soup or stew with a salad

DESSERT:
Maple Caramelized Apples (page 149) with or without a little yogurt, or a scoop of vanilla frozen yogurt or ice cream

SNACKS (midmorning or midafternoon; always optional):
an apple; ½ cup of leftover Almond Butter and Strawberry Breakfast Smoothie; some roasted nuts; tea

Day 4

BREAKFAST:

Make It: Whole Grain French Toast (1 or 2 slices) with Fresh Papaya (page 146) or other fresh fruit

Sort of Make It: Lightly buttered whole grain toast (1 or 2 slices) with a slice of cheese and fresh fruit (or leftover Maple Caramelized Apples)

LUNCH:

Make It: Pear, Watercress, and Blue Cheese Salad (page 158)

Don't Make It: Leftover Spicy Chickpea and Tomato Stew with Spinach

Don't Make It: Lightly dressed salad (sprinkle with olive oil, lemon, salt) with a fist-size serving of a protein (tofu, chicken, cheese, nuts, etc.)

DINNER:

Make It: Roasted Halibut with Zucchini and Mint Pesto (page 204) and ½ cup brown rice

Sort of Make It: Toasted Broccoli with Cheddar (page 167; we promise, this is really almost like not cooking at all) and 1 slice of whole grain bread

DESSERT:

What will scratch your itch? Or fruit and a cookie (1 or 2 depending on the size)

SNACKS (midmorning or midafternoon; always optional):

½ cup yogurt with some fruit; Retro Broiled Grapefruit (page 150) or plain grapefruit; tea; pineapple or papaya; a small handful of nuts (with or without a few squares of dark chocolate)

WEEK 1

Day 5

BREAKFAST:

Make It: Banana and Kiwi Smoothie (1 cup) (page 153)

Don't Make It: Yogurt and cut-up fruit with a sprinkling of nuts if you'd like the "crunch"

LUNCH:

Make It: Prosciutto, Mozzarella, Breadsticks, Cherry Tomatoes, and Celery Sticks (page 178)

Don't Make It: Ditto. You can probably buy something like it at a nearby food shop.

Don't Make It: Leftover halibut over salad-bar field greens (sprinkled with olive oil, lemon, and salt)

DINNER:

Sort of Make It: Pad Thai (ordered in) with Sauteed Broccoli with Red Pepper Flakes (page 217))

Sort of Make It: A big serving of Seared Artichoke Hearts with Pecorino and Basil (page 215) over whole wheat pasta (½ cup to 1 cup uncooked/person)

DESSERT:

Mango and a smallish piece of shortbread or just mango or just shortbread, depending on your mood

SNACKS (midmorning or midafternoon; always optional):
Tea (surprised?); a banana; an orange (plain or gussied up with a little olive oil, salt, and fresh herbs); one chocolate-covered pretzel or a few almonds; some leftover Somewhat-Lighter Baba Ganouj with Yogurt on pita or a slice of pumpernickel

WEEK 1

Day 6

BREAKFAST:

Make It: Muesli with Raisins, Nuts, and Apple or Pear (1 cup of muesli, not counting the fruit) (page 147)

Sort of Make It: Oatmeal with fresh fruit and ¼ cup milk

LUNCH:

Make It: Quick Kale and White Bean Soup (1 cup; page 199) and Tomato-Herb Salad with Goat Cheese (page 164)

Don't Make It: The (veggie or bean) soup-and-salad special (dress salad lightly)

Don't Make It: Leftover pad Thai and Sauteed Broccoli with Red Pepper Flakes, 3 or 4 apricots or other fresh fruit

DINNER:

Make it: Roasted Chicken Breast with Rosemary Apples (page 208) (or substitute salmon for the chicken) and ½ cup Israeli or regular or whole wheat couscous or bulgur

Don't Make It: Take-out roasted chicken, a salad, and a whole wheat tortilla

DESSERT:

Whole Wheat Cherry Scones (page 148) with ½ cup yogurt and fresh strawberries (if you feel like baking) or fresh fruit and/or a small cookie (1 or 2, depending on the size)

SNACKS (midmorning or midafternoon; always optional): Tea (still surprised?); honeydew (cut up from the deli); Addictive Spiced Popcorn (page 185)

WEEK 1

Day 7

BREAKFAST:

Make It: Retro Broiled (or half of a plain) Grapefruit
(page 150), a slice of whole grain toast, and a poached egg (you
can leave off any one of these three elements for a perfectly
fine breakfast)

LUNCH:

Make It: Caesar Salad to Die (But Not Get Fat) For
(page 192) with leftover chicken (4 to 6 ounces or a fist-size
portion) or 4 to 6 shrimp (from the freezer, just run them under
cold water to defrost)

Don't Make It: Sandwich (turkey, roast beef, ham, cheese,
grilled seitan) on whole grain bread (hold the mayo) and a small
green salad (if you like, try having half the sandwich now and
half later for snack) (*Note*: If you can't get the sandwich into
your mouth because it's stuffed so full, unstuff it and throw
away the excess meat or cheese or save for tomorrow.)

DINNER:

Make It: London Broil with Caramelized Pineapple (page 210)

Don't Make It: Go out. Don't finish everything on your plate.
Take it home if you think you'll eat it for lunch tomorrow.

DESSERT:

Roasted Peaches with Black Pepper, Brown Sugar, and
Balsamic (page 188) or fresh fruit and/or a cookie (1 or
2, depending on the size)

SNACKS (midmorning or midafternoon; always optional): You
decide, but if you made scones, there's probably still
one around.

WEEK 1

WEEK TWO

Day 8

BREAKFAST:

Yogurt (1 cup) with leftover roasted peaches (or fresh peaches or other fruit) and a slice of whole grain toast (or not)

LUNCH:

Sort of Make It: Leftover steak sandwich on whole grain bread with ½ cup of (leftover) white bean and chicory or other vegetable-rich soup

Don't Make It: 1 cup soup (either the white bean and chicory or something you've bought), a lightly dressed salad with or without a whole grain roll

DINNER:

Make It: Turkey or Pork Sausage with Spicy Sauteed Broccoli Rabe (page 209) and brown rice or ½ cup whole grain pasta

Sort of Make It: Seared Sashimi à la Nobu (page 226) with Japanese vegetables (order in the sashimi and vegetables) and ½ cup brown rice

DESSERT:

A reasonable square of chocolate (bar sizes vary, but no matter the size, stick to half or less—unless it's a "fun size") with or without fresh watermelon (or other fruit)

SNACKS (midmorning or midafternoon; always optional): banana; do we need to say tea?; spinach-and-yogurt dip or a few slices of avocado on rye crisps or whole grain crackers; a small handful of nuts

Day 9

BREAKFAST:

Make It (maybe): Muesli with Raisins, Nuts, and Apple or Pear (page 147)

Don't Make It: 1 cup of whole grain cereal with fat-free soymilk or rice milk and banana and/or berries

LUNCH:

Make It: Tuna and Cucumber Salad with Olives (page 170) and an apple

Don't Make It: Italian tuna salad (no mayo) from a gourmet shop or roasted/grilled salmon from a salad bar over lightly dressed greens or some other protein (4 to 6 ounces of chicken, cheese, nuts, tofu), an apple

DINNER:

Make It: Roasted Eggplant, Peppers, Onions, and Cherry Tomatoes with an Egg on Top (page 194). Don't want the egg? Mix in some tofu.

Don't Make It: Order in Steamed Mixed Vegetables with Asian Dipping Sauce (page 222) or Blue Cheese (page 223)

DESSERT:

Berries and/or a (half) slice of pound cake from your favorite bakery

SNACKS (midmorning or midafternoon; always optional):
½ cup yogurt with or without banana; tea, of course; a whole grain roll with a small pat of butter; Retro Broiled Grapefruit (page 150) or a piece of citrus fruit

Day 10

BREAKFAST:

Make It: One or two eggs any way you like with one slice of whole grain lightly buttered toast

Sort of Make It: Are there any scones left? Have one with either ½ cup yogurt or an egg.

LUNCH:

Make It: Watermelon, Feta, and Olive Salad (page 177) with flatbread/pita

Don't Make It: Leftover Roasted Eggplant, Peppers, Onions, and Cherry Tomatoes sprinkled with (up to) ½ cup cubed mozzarella cheese

DINNER:

Make It: Seared Garlicky Squid or Shrimp over Mixed Greens (page 206) (or whatever fish dish you please if you don't want shrimp or squid)

Don't Make It: Cold Sesame Noodles and Cucumber Salad (page 225). Have about 1 cup noodles with unlimited cucumbers.

DESSERT:

Fresh fruit and ½ cup yogurt or vanilla ice cream (1 small scoop) or 1 scoop of whatever kind of ice cream

SNACKS (midmorning or midafternoon; always optional):
Chocolate (a few squares, preferably dark); a tomato cut up and sprinkled with salt and a little lemon juice; have you considered a big mug of tea with milk?

Day 11

BREAKFAST:

Make It: Almond Butter and Strawberry Breakfast Smoothie (page 152)

Don't Make It: 1 cup yogurt with fruit

LUNCH:

Make It: Bulgur Salad with Scallions, Parsley, Cucumber, and Tomatoes (page 176) with a pear or other piece of fruit

Don't Make It: Ditto. Is there Middle Eastern takeout nearby?

Don't Make It: Leftover Cold Sesame Noodles and Cucumber Salad (1 cup) and a pear

DINNER:

Make It: Seared Tuna with Parsley and Dried Tomato Salad (page 203)

Don't Make It: Take-out roasted or grilled chicken or fish with plenty of vegetables

DESSERT:

You know what you have and what you want.

SNACKS (midmorning or midafternoon; always optional):

You can guess what we'd suggest—any big ideas? Some Half-and-Half Guacamole (page 184) with carrot sticks? Watermelon? ½ cup of Moroccan Carrot Salad with Coriander and Cashews (page 172)? A small bowl of edamame?

Day 12

BREAKFAST:

Make It: Whole Grain French Toast with Fresh Papaya (or other fruit) (page 146)

Sort of Make It: Lightly buttered whole grain toast (1 or 2 slices), a slice of cheese, fresh fruit

LUNCH:

Make It: Chicken Salad (use leftover chicken) with Roasted Red Peppers (page 171) over greens

Don't Make It: Hummus (about ½ cup) with pita and greens

DINNER:

Make It: Roasted Tofu with Shiitake, Soy, and Ginger over Baby Spinach (page 197) with boiled soba noodles or ½ cup brown rice

Sort of Make It: Fast Winter Squash Soup with Lime (page 213), a hunk of bread, a little butter, and some cheese

DESSERT:

Shortbread and/or papaya and/or …?

SNACKS (midmorning or midafternoon; always optional):
Watermelon (cut up from the deli); an apple with cheese; ½ cup of yogurt with some banana; some tea!

Day 13

BREAKFAST:

Make It: Oatmeal (1 cup) with fresh fruit

Don't Make It: Whole grain cereal (1 cup) with skim/soy/rice milk and fresh fruit

LUNCH:

Make It: Tuna and Cucumber Salad with Olives (page 170)

Don't Make It: Leftover Roasted Tofu with Shiitake, Soy, and Ginger over Baby Spinach, plus an apple

Don't Make It: Sushi rolls (veggie and/or fish, 1 or 2 depending on size) and edamame

DINNER:

Make It: Roasted Chicken Breasts with Rosemary Apples (page 208)

Don't Make It: Order in pad Thai

DESSERT:

You have any of that ice cream around? Have 1 small scoop.

SNACKS (midmorning or midafternoon; always optional):

1 slice of whole grain toast with almond butter (less than 1 tablespoon); banana; pear; some nuts; tea (we had to say it)

Day 14

BREAKFAST:

Make It: Banana and Kiwi (or other fruit) Smoothie (page 153)

Don't Make It: Yogurt (1 cup) and fruit

LUNCH:

Make It: Moroccan Carrot Salad with Coriander and Cashews (page 172), whole wheat pita, and 2 or 3 fresh figs

Don't Make It: Feel like a sandwich? Get it on whole grain bread, hold the mayo, nothing fried inside.

DINNER:

Make It: Pan-Seared Red Snapper with Chunky Cherry Tomato Sauce and Garlic (page 205)

Don't Make It: Go out. Don't finish everything on your plate. Bring leftovers home if you think you'll eat them tomorrow.

DESSERT:

You must know by now!

SNACKS:

You pick. Choose from one of the previous days if you need some ideas.

A Brief and Basic Nutrition Glossary

Antioxidant

An antioxidant is any substance that slows or stops the destructive effects of oxidation. Outside the body, for example, oxidation causes silver to tarnish. Inside the body, molecules called free radicals (they're produced by normal metabolic processes) oxidize cells. Over time, those oxidized cells can lead to diseases such as cancer. Antioxidants neutralize free radicals; they include vitamins A, C, and E, some of the B vitamins, beta-carotene, and selenium (and flavonoids).

B vitamins

Also called B-complex vitamins or B-vitamin complex, these are a group of eight water-soluble vitamins that your body must get through food or dietary supplements because the body doesn't manufacture them. B vitamins aid in cell development, convert food into energy, and help maintain healthy vision, skin, and muscle tissue. They're found in foods such as grains, cereals, green leafy vegetables, citrus fruits, dried beans and peas, cauliflower, eggs, liver, and yeast. The B vitamins include B_1 (thiamin), B_2 (riboflavin), B_3 (niacin), B_5 (pantothenic acid), B_6 (pyridoxine and pyridoxamine), B_7 (biotin), B_9 (folic acid), and B_{12} (cobalamin).

Beta-carotene

This is the stuff that makes carrots orange and leafy greens very dark green. We're talking about foods such as spinach, kale, watercress, sweet potatoes, broccoli, cantaloupe, and oranges. The deeper the color, the more plentiful the beta-carotene. The body converts beta-carotene into vitamin A, which helps with cell division, vision, bone growth, and reproduction. Vitamin A also helps regulate the immune system and may protect against cancer and heart disease.

Body Mass Index

Body Mass Index (BMI) is a measurement of weight relative to height. The USDA considers a BMI of between 18.5 and 24.9 healthy. If you like to do math, you can calculate your BMI by dividing your weight in pounds by your height in inches squared. Then, multiply that number by 703. Or you can use the online calculator from the National Heart, Blood, and Lung Institute at www.nhlbisupport.com/bmi/bmicalc.htm.

BODY MASS INDEX TABLE

HEIGHT IN INCHES / BODY WEIGHT (POUNDS)

BMI	19	20	21	22	23	24	25	26	27	28	29	30	31	32	33	34	35	36	37	38	39	40
	NORMAL						OVERWEIGHT					OBESE										
58	91	96	100	105	110	115	119	124	129	134	138	143	148	153	158	162	167	172	177	181	186	191
59	94	99	104	109	114	119	124	128	133	138	143	148	153	158	163	168	173	178	183	188	193	198
60	97	102	107	112	118	123	128	133	138	143	148	153	158	163	168	174	179	184	189	194	199	204
61	100	106	111	116	122	127	132	137	143	148	153	158	164	169	174	180	185	190	195	201	206	211
62	104	109	115	120	126	131	136	142	147	153	158	164	169	175	180	186	191	196	202	207	213	218
63	107	113	118	124	130	135	141	146	152	158	163	169	175	180	186	191	197	203	208	214	220	225
64	110	116	122	128	134	140	145	151	157	163	169	174	180	186	192	197	204	209	215	221	227	232
65	114	120	126	132	138	144	150	156	162	168	174	180	186	192	198	204	210	216	222	228	234	240
66	118	124	130	136	142	148	155	161	167	173	179	186	192	198	204	210	216	223	229	235	241	247
67	121	127	134	140	146	153	159	166	172	178	185	191	198	204	211	217	223	230	236	242	249	255
68	125	131	138	144	151	158	164	171	177	184	190	197	203	210	216	223	230	236	243	249	256	262
69	128	135	142	149	155	162	169	176	182	189	196	203	209	216	223	230	236	243	250	257	263	270
70	132	139	146	153	160	167	174	181	188	195	202	209	216	222	229	236	243	250	257	264	271	278
71	136	143	150	157	165	172	179	186	193	200	208	215	222	229	236	243	250	257	265	272	279	286
72	140	147	154	162	169	177	184	191	199	206	213	221	228	235	242	250	258	265	272	279	287	294
73	144	151	159	166	174	182	189	197	204	212	219	227	235	242	250	257	265	272	280	288	295	302
74	148	155	163	171	179	186	194	202	210	218	225	233	241	249	256	264	272	280	287	295	303	311
75	152	160	168	176	184	192	200	208	216	224	232	240	248	256	264	272	279	287	295	303	311	319
76	156	164	172	180	189	197	205	213	221	230	238	246	254	263	271	279	287	295	304	312	320	328

Source: Adapted from Clinical Guidelines on the Identification, Evaluation, and Treatment of Overweight and Obesity in Adults: The Evidence Report.

Calcium

Calcium is the most plentiful mineral in your body. In addition to keeping bones and teeth strong, it helps with muscle contraction, the smooth functioning of the heart, and the secretion of hormones and enzymes. Women of childbearing age (19 to 50) are advised to consume about 1,000 milligrams of calcium per day. Not everyone gets that much. According to the Continuing Survey of Food Intakes by Individuals, 78 percent of women don't consume enough calcium. Dairy foods have calcium, as do broccoli, rhubarb, almonds, blackstrap molasses, calcium-fortified orange juice, calcium-fortified tofu and soymilk, and leafy green vegetables such as bok choy and dandelion greens.

Calorie

A calorie is a measurement of the amount of energy it takes to increase the temperature of one gram of water one degree centigrade. To lose weight you need to use more calories in a day than you eat.

Carbohydrates

These are a primary source of energy for the body. Carbs are found in grains such as rice, wheat, and barley; potatoes; fruits and vegetables; and (in case you need a reminder) wine, beer, and soda. Everyone needs carbohydrates from produce and whole grains for vitamins, minerals, and fiber (which is also a carbohydrate). No one needs carbohydrates from white bread and cake and cookies because they have no extra nutrients— they were all stripped away in the milling process. You may need other things from those foods, of course (such as pleasure), but you're not eating them because they're good for you.

Cholesterol

The liver makes cholesterol, which is a waxy substance that helps in the formation of cell membranes and some hormones. Even though we need cholesterol, too much of it can build up in arteries. When enough cholesterol clumps together, it forms plaque, which can narrow an artery or cause blood clots. The consequences can be devastating: heart attacks and strokes.

There are both good and bad types of cholesterol. Low-density lipoproteins (LDL) are the bad kind that can build up on artery walls. High-density lipoproteins (HDL) are good; they take LDL cholesterol out of the blood and return it to the liver for elimination.

Fat

Even though we've been trained to find it scary, fat is necessary for a well-functioning body. Fat builds cell membranes, keeps our hair and skin healthy, insulates our body, protects our organs from shock, and keeps us warm. Some vitamins—such as vitamins A, D, E, and K—are fat soluble, which means they need fat to be digested and used. There are several kinds of fats:

The very good fats: monounsaturated. These lower LDL (bad) cholesterol levels and raise HDL (good) cholesterol levels. Sources include nuts, avocados, olives and olive oil, peanut oil, and canola oil.

The still-good fats: polyunsaturated. These include the well-known omega-3 essential fatty acids (the body doesn't produce them, but it needs them). Polyunsaturated fats are in nuts, seeds, soybean and corn oils, and cold-water fatty fish such as salmon and tuna.

The bad fats: saturated. All fats are saturated (as you can tell from the names of the other fats). But when a fat is just saturated (and not polyunsaturated or monounsaturated), it will tend to raise bad (LDL) cholesterol levels. Animal fat and dairy are full of saturated fats. Eat foods with saturated fats in moderation.

The really bad fats: trans fats. Trans fats are bad. The body doesn't need them, and they cause heart disease. When you read food labels, look out for "partially hydrogenated oils" and "hydrogenated oils" because these are trans fats. Avoid them.

Fiber

Fiber is a carbohydrate in fruits, vegetables, plants, and legumes. You can't digest it, and this is exactly why it's good for you. As fiber passes through your digestive tract, it takes partially digested food along for a ride. This slows the process of digestion and keeps you feeling full longer. Fiber helps reduce the risk of heart disease, type 2 diabetes, and diverticular disease. Fiber also keeps you "regular," and we know you know what that means.

Fiber is commonly broken down into two categories: soluble and insoluble. Both aid in digestion and the prevention of heart disease. Soluble fiber is in foods like oatmeal, nuts, legumes (beans, lentils, dried peas), apples, bananas, broccoli, yams, strawberries, pears, and blueberries. Insoluble fiber is found in whole grains like barley, brown rice, bulgur, and whole grain cereal; it's also in veggies like green beans, cauliflower, celery, and the skin of tomatoes.

Glycemic Index and glycemic load

When people talk about carbohydrates, they used to talk about complex carbs and simple carbs—but that's so over. Now people talk about the Glycemic Index (GI). The GI measures how quickly and how high blood sugar spikes after eating 50 grams of a specific food. The GI of white bread is 100, an apple's is 55.

But because nothing is simple, a food's glycemic load is just as important to consider as its GI. Glycemic load is a number that multiplies a food's GI by the amount of carbs in an individual serving. Glycemic load gives you a better sense of how an individual serving of a specific food might affect you and your blood sugar. Take the carrot, for example. It has a relatively high GI of 113, but that index number is based on eating 50 grams of the carbohydrate in the food. To eat 50 grams of carbs in carrots, you'd have to eat about one and a half pounds of carrots! But what if you only eat half a cup? You'd be taking on a glycemic load of about 10, which is low. See?

For a searchable database of foods and their GI and load numbers, go online to www.glycemicindex.com.

Macronutrients

Macronutrients are those nutrients that give the body the great majority of its metabolic energy. Carbohydrates, proteins, and fat are the three primary macronutrients for humans.

Metabolism

This is the process by which chemical compounds, such as vitamins, phytonutrients, and calories, are modified by a living organism and cells. In other words, it's the way the body turns calories into energy.

Minerals

Minerals—such as calcium, magnesium, potassium, selenium, zinc, sodium, and iron—are inorganic substances that we need in small amounts for our bodies to function.

Phytochemicals

Also called phytonutrients, these are usually plant-based substances that the body doesn't need for normal, basic functioning but that are good for you nonetheless. Most phytonutrients are antioxidants; they help fight heart disease, reduce the risk of cancer, and boost immunity. Foods that are rich in phytochemicals include soy, tomato, broccoli, garlic, citrus, watermelon, blueberries, sweet potatoes, and garlic.

Protein

Protein gives us energy, builds and repairs body tissue, and produces enzymes and hormones. Foods have either complete or incomplete proteins. Complete proteins have the nine essential amino acids that the body needs to build protein but does not produce; they're found in meat, fish, eggs, dairy, and soy. Incomplete proteins are low or lacking in at least one of these nine amino acids; they're found in grains, nuts, and legumes.

Vitamins

A vitamin is an organic molecule that the body needs in small amounts to stay healthy. Vitamins dissolve either in water (water soluble) or fat (fat soluble). The body processes vitamins most efficiently when they come from whole foods as opposed to dietary supplements.

Index

Recipe Index